ENDOMORPH DIET AND EXERCISE PLAN

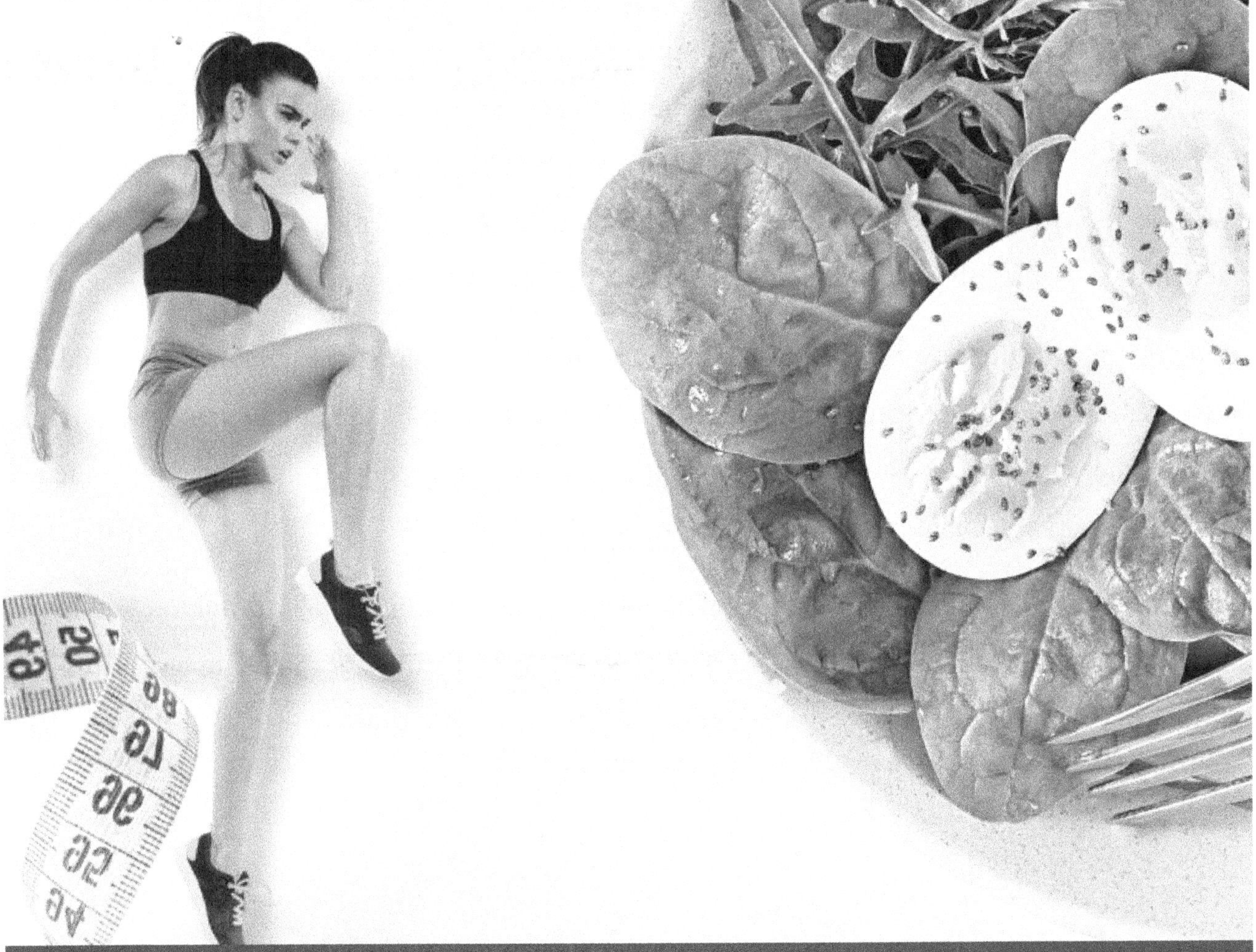

CLAUDIA ADKINS

LEGAL DISCLAIMER

This book serves as educational and entertainment material and is not a substitute for professional medical advice or treatment. While the information presented here is sourced from reliable outlets to the best of the Author's knowledge, accuracy cannot be guaranteed. The Author cannot be held responsible for any errors or omissions. It is advisable to consult a medical professional before implementing any remedies or techniques suggested in this book.

By utilizing the information provided, you agree to absolve the Author and Publisher of any liability for damages, expenses, or legal fees arising from the application of the advice contained herein. This disclaimer encompasses any damages or injuries resulting directly or indirectly from the use of the information presented, regardless of the cause of action.

You acknowledge and assume all risks associated with the utilization of the information within this book. It is recommended to consult with a qualified medical practitioner to ensure suitability and safety before engaging in any program outlined herein.

About the Author

Claudia Adkins' journey into the world of health and nutrition didn't start with a textbook; it began in the heart of her kitchen. As a cook with a deep passion for creating delicious meals, Claudia found true fulfillment when she discovered the profound impact food has on our well-being. This revelation led her to become a certified nutritionist and, ultimately, an advocate for health and happiness for everyone.

Unlike some diet gurus, Claudia's path wasn't one of effortless thinness or a lifetime spent memorizing calorie charts. Like many of us, she has grappled with understanding her own body and navigating the often-confusing world of dietary advice. As an endomorph herself, Claudia understands the unique challenges endomorphs face – the slower metabolism, the constant battle against cravings, and the frustration of feeling like the odds are stacked against them.

That's why Claudia created "The Endomorph Diet and Exercise Plan." It's not just a collection of recipes or a rigid set of rules. It's a roadmap to a healthier, happier you, built on the foundation of her personal experience, culinary expertise, and years of nutritional research.

Claudia's approach is all about empowerment and sustainability. She guides you on how to fuel your body with delicious, nourishing food that satisfies your cravings while supporting your unique metabolic needs. She delves into exercise strategies that fit your lifestyle and preferences, helping you build muscle and boost your metabolism for lasting results.

But most importantly, Claudia's journey is about reclaiming a sense of joy and connection with your body. She teaches you to cultivate a mindful approach to eating, celebrate the power of movement, and discover the true meaning of well-being.

This isn't just about shedding pounds; it's about embracing a vibrant, energetic life. So, join Claudia in the kitchen, embark on a mindful movement practice, and start this journey of transformation together. You've got this, and Claudia is here to guide you every step of the way.

Ready to unlock your inner wellness warrior? Dive into "The Endomorph Diet and Exercise Plan" by Claudia Adkins and let's get cooking!

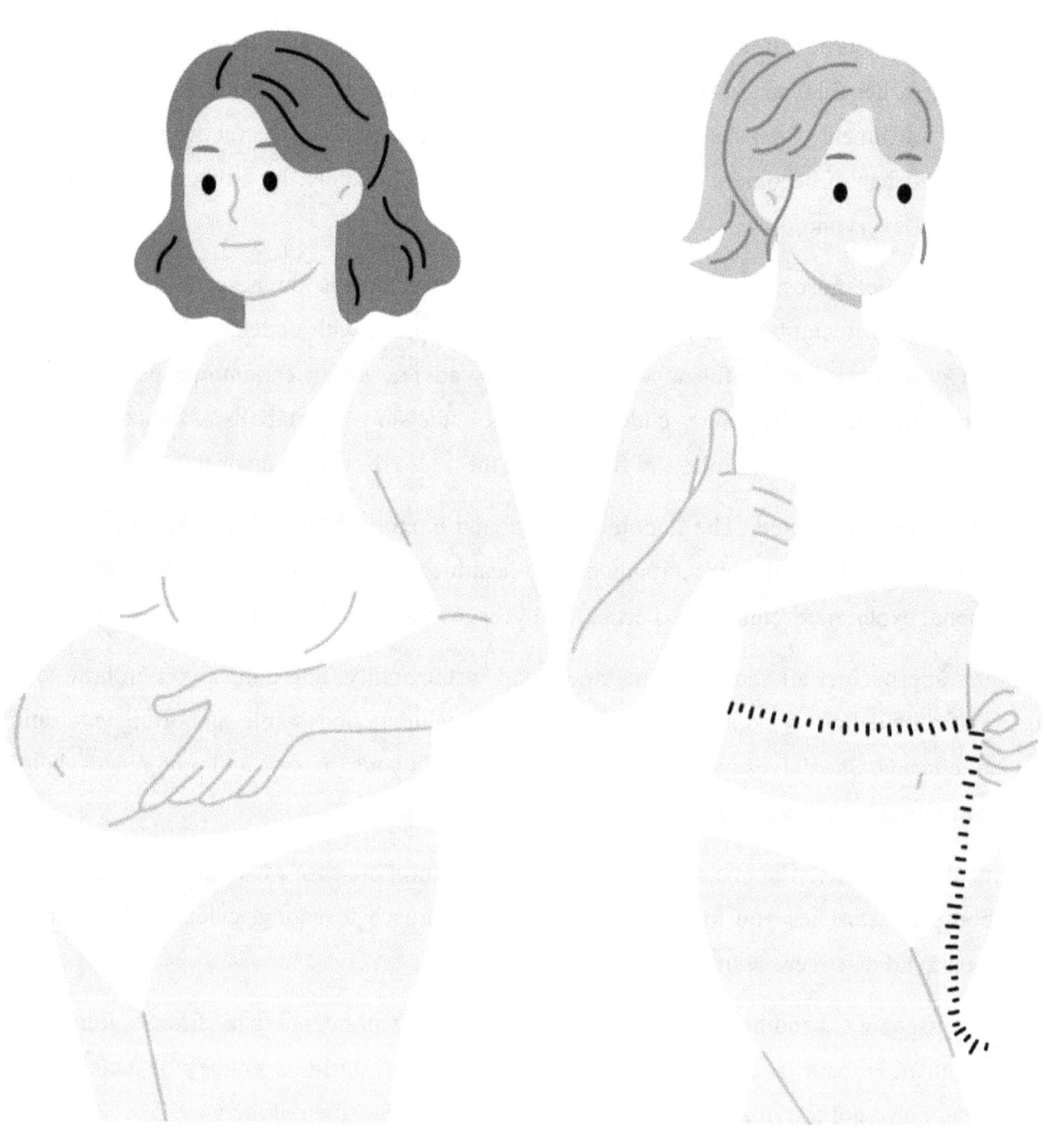

Table of Contents

Introduction

Welcome to the journey of discovering and valuing your body type to reach your best possible state of health and well-being. This book will walk you through the process of changing your lifestyle in a fun and sustainable manner. We highlight the endomorph body type, which finds it difficult to lose weight and tends to gain it readily. After learning about your body's requirements, you can develop a diet and exercise regimen that suits your unique demands to live a happier, more energetic life.

As a cook, nutritionist, and advocate for health and well-being, I have a strong belief in enabling people—especially women—to make decisions that will help them achieve their health objectives. You'll get the information, resources, and motivation you need from this book to take charge of your health. We will delve into the science behind body types, metabolism, and the importance of individualized diet and exercise plans. One step at a time, together, we will walk the path to a healthier you.

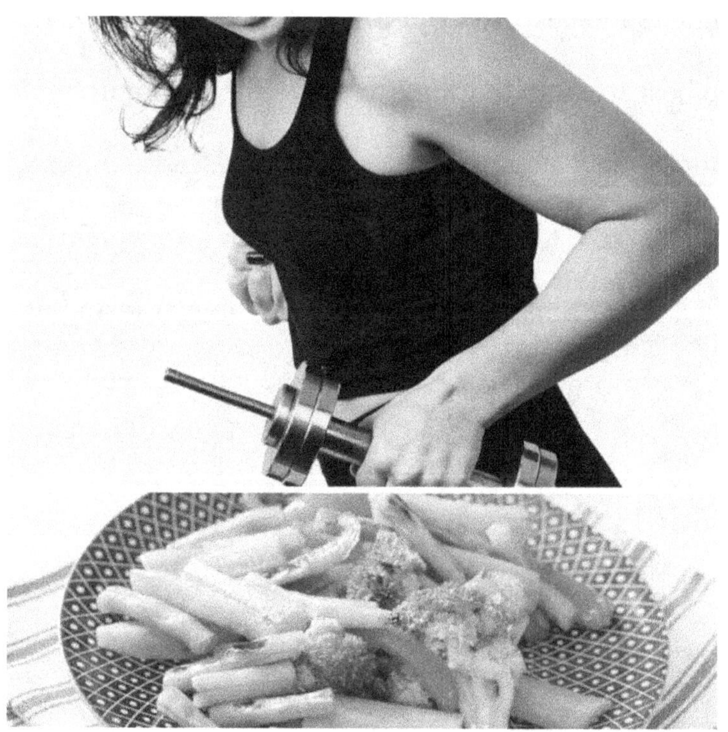

Chapter 1 - What Exactly is an Endomorph?

Understanding Body Types

During the 1940s, Dr. William Sheldon developed the concept of somatotypes or body types. Ectomorph, mesomorph, and endomorph were his three basic body types for humans. In relation to metabolism, muscular growth, and weight gain, every body type has unique traits and tendencies. Generally speaking, an ectomorph is long and slender, has a quick metabolism, and struggles to put on weight or muscle. Conversely, mesomorphs are built more athletically and muscularly, grow muscle more quickly, and have a metabolism that is modestly quick. Endomorphs, the subject of this book, are more likely to accumulate fat, are frequently rounder in shape, and may have slower metabolisms.

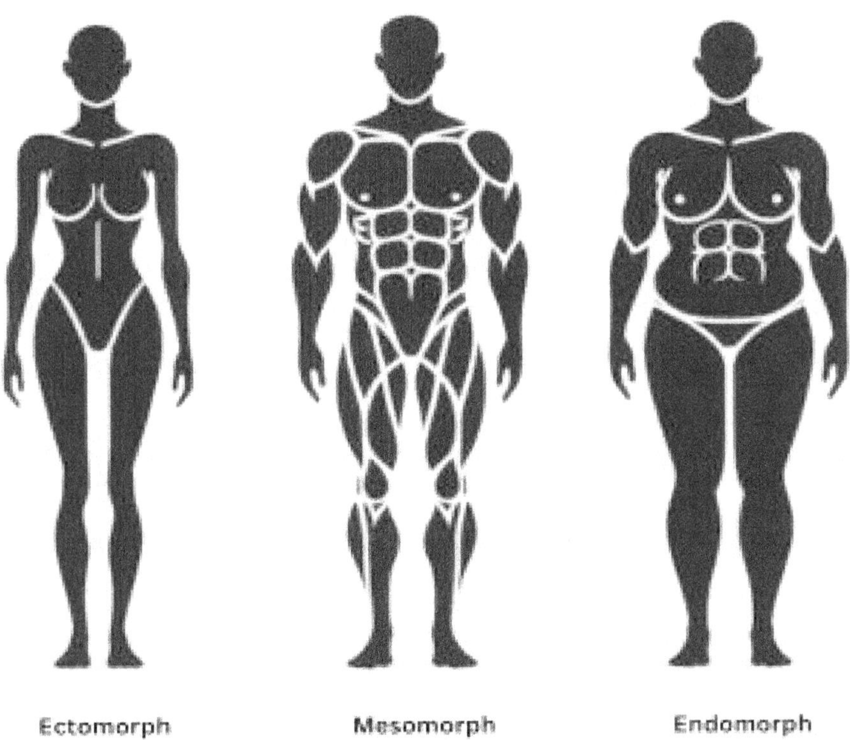

Physical Characteristics of Endomorphs

Endomorphs frequently share several identifying morphological traits:

- Greater Body Fat Percentage: Generally speaking, endomorphs have a larger body fat percentage, particularly in the thighs, hips, and midsection.
- Rounder Physique: Compared to being angular and slim, the body shape is usually round and soft.
- Bones and Joints: Endomorphs typically have bigger joints and bone structures.
- Easy Fat Storage: Endomorphs store fat more easily because of metabolic variances, making it more difficult to lose weight.
- Muscle Mass: Although endomorphs can develop muscle somewhat quickly, if improperly controlled, this is frequently accompanied by an increased fat mass.

Endomorph Comparisons to Other Body Types Recognizing the variations among the three body types helps to emphasize the special requirements and benefits of each. Because of their rapid metabolism and weight gain issues, ectomorphs need a high-calorie diet and a concentration on strength training to gain muscle. Mesomorphs do best with a well-balanced diet and workout regimen that emphasizes preserving their naturally muscular physique.

To effectively maintain their weight, endomorphs must, however, approach diet and exercise more strategically. Their slowed metabolism necessitates a diet high in low-calorie, nutrient-dense foods. Exercises combining strength and cardio also help increase metabolism and encourage fat loss while maintaining muscular mass.

Endomorph Myths Debunked

Endomorphs, the naturally "curvy" body type, often face a barrage of misconceptions. Let's tackle some of the most common myths and empower you to embrace your unique strengths!

Myth #1: Building Muscle is an Endomorph's Kryptonite

Truth bomb: Genetics do influence muscle growth, but appearance isn't the sole predictor. Consistent strength training, regardless of body type, can build muscle and boost metabolism. Don't be fooled by the initial physique – hidden potential awaits!

Myth #2: There's a "Magic Food List" for Endomorphs

While some dietary approaches might work better for you than others, there's no one-size-fits-all solution. The key is finding a sustainable, balanced eating plan you can stick with. Focus on whole foods, prioritize protein, and don't demonize specific ingredients.

Myth #3: Endomorphs Lack Willpower

This myth is not only insensitive but untrue. Body size doesn't define self-control. Focus on building healthy habits and celebrate progress, not perfection. Remember, consistency trumps perfection in the long run.

Myth #4: Endomorphs are Destined for Poor Health

A higher body fat percentage is a characteristic of endomorphs, but it doesn't automatically equal poor health. Many endomorphs live active, healthy lives. Focus on overall well-being through a balanced lifestyle, not just weight loss.

Myth #5: Limited Athletic Options for Endomorphs

Forget the myth that certain activities are off-limits! Endomorphs can excel in a variety of sports and exercises. Find activities you enjoy – yoga, swimming, weightlifting – the options are endless! The most important factor? Find activities you'll stick with and that make you feel great.

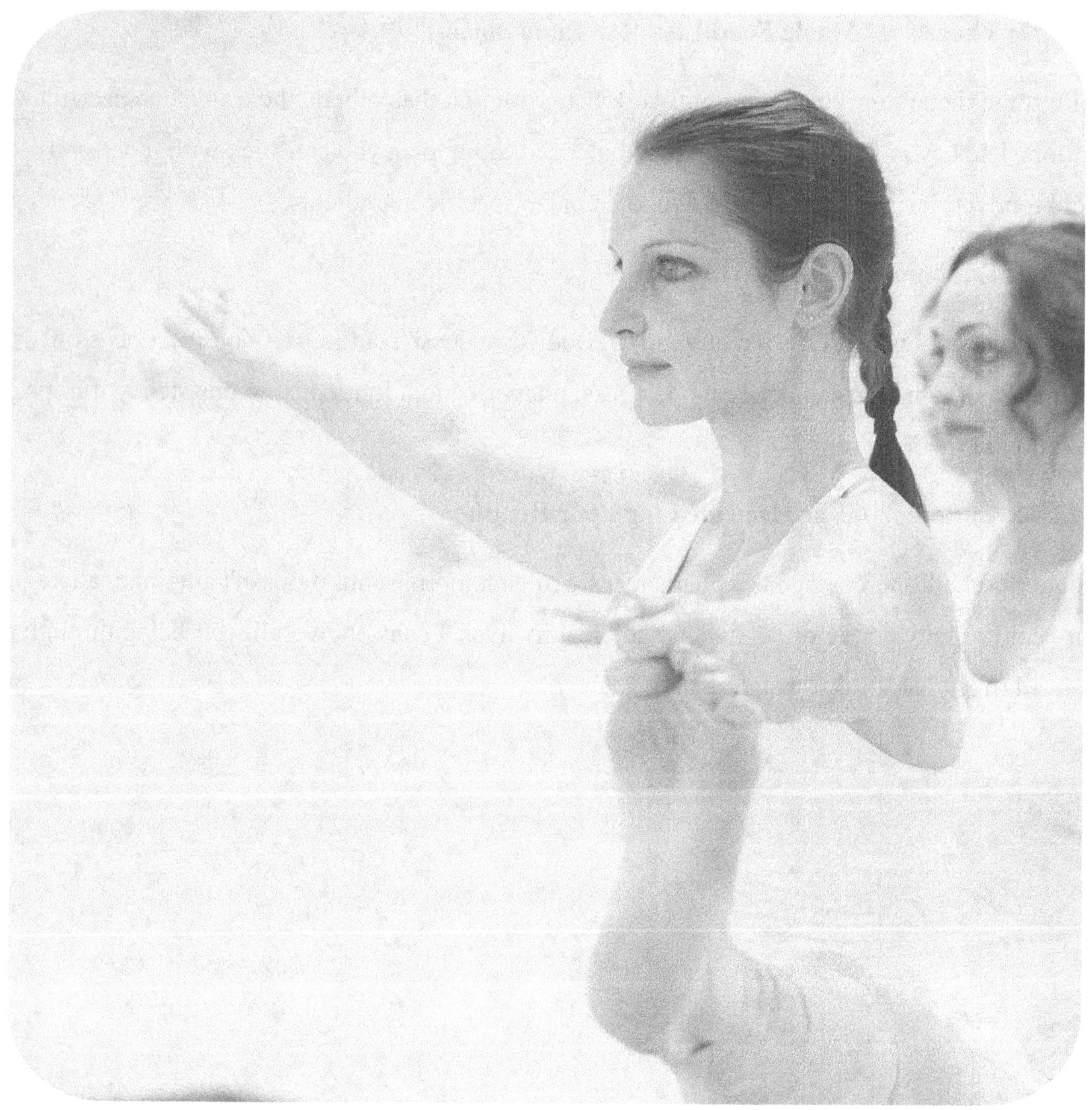

Chapter 2 - Start Up Your Body's Metabolism

Fat Burning and Body Metabolism

The body turns food into energy through a process called metabolism. It includes every chemical reaction your cells go through to keep you alive. For endomorphs, efficient weight control depends on knowing their metabolism.

There are three main components of metabolism:

BMR: The number of calories required by your body to sustain fundamental physiological processes like breathing, circulation, and cell creation is known as your basal metabolic rate or BMR. Comparatively speaking to ectomorphs and mesomorphs, endomorphs frequently have a lower BMR.

TEF, or thermal effect of food, is the amount of energy needed for nutrition, digestion, absorption, and elimination. This effect accounts for about 10% of your daily calorie intake.

Physical activity: This involves any movement, from daily tasks like walking and housework to exercise. To increase their total caloric expenditure, endomorphs must become more physically active.

Endomorph: Metabolic Features

Because of specific metabolic traits, endomorphs approach diet and exercise differently:

Slower Metabolism: Because endomorphs naturally burn fewer calories at rest, gaining weight is simpler and losing it more difficult.

Insulin Sensitivity: Higher fat storage and trouble controlling blood sugar levels can result from endomorphs' increased susceptibility to insulin resistance.

Hormonal Impacts: In endomorphs, imbalances in hormones like leptin and ghrelin, which control hunger and satiety, can cause cravings and increased appetite.

Knowing these features facilitates customizing a diet and exercise regimen that optimizes metabolic efficiency and promotes weight loss.

The Importance of a Healthy Weight

Remaining at a healthy weight is essential to general health and the avoidance of chronic illnesses including heart disease, diabetes, and several malignancies. Reaching and keeping a healthy weight requires endomorphs to:

- Balanced nutrition is the emphasis of a diet high in whole, unprocessed foods that supply vital nutrients without adding too many calories.
- Regular Exercise: Increasing metabolic rate and promoting fat reduction by including strength and cardiovascular training activities.
- Lifestyle Adjustments: Taking up long-term weight management-supporting, sustainable habits including stress management, enough sleep, and mindful eating.

Insulin in Endomorphs

For endomorphs, understanding how insulin impacts the body is essential, as they often face challenges related to insulin resistance. This section will explain what insulin is, its roles in the body, the causes of insulin resistance, and practical strategies for managing it.

Understanding Insulin Resistance

Insulin, a hormone produced by your pancreas, acts like a key, unlocking the door for glucose (sugar) from food to enter your cells and provide energy. However, sometimes these cellular "doors" become resistant to insulin's message. This is called insulin resistance.

Endomorphs, known for their slower metabolisms and higher predisposition to storing fat, often have a trickier relationship with insulin. Their bodies tend to be more efficient at converting carbohydrates into sugar, which can lead to blood sugar spikes. Over time, this can overwhelm the body's ability to manage insulin effectively, potentially increasing the risk of insulin resistance and related conditions like type 2 diabetes.

To address this, endomorphs can benefit from dietary strategies that promote healthy blood sugar levels. This often involves limiting processed, refined carbohydrates that cause rapid sugar spikes. Instead, prioritizing protein and healthy fats helps promote satiety and provide sustained energy. Think lean meats, fish, eggs, legumes, nuts, avocados, and olive oil – these nutrient-rich options can become your allies in managing insulin and supporting your overall health.

Managing Insulin Resistance

Healthy diet

An endomorph should revamp their diet to overcome insulin resistance. Give up processed meals, refined carbohydrates, and sweets since they exacerbate insulin resistance and cause blood sugar rises. Rather, concentrate on packing your plate full of entire, nutrient-dense meals. Consider lean meats, fruits, veggies, and healthy fats. Remember to incorporate low-GI foods like legumes and vegetables, which assist in maintaining stable blood sugar levels by releasing sugar gradually. According to research, endomorphs may benefit from cutting back on total carbohydrates, so explore to determine what feels good for you. Ultimately, the secret to losing weight is to start with a small calorie deficit because endomorphs have slower metabolisms. Your body needs this shortfall to provide the right conditions to burn fat.

Regular Exercise

Do weight training as well as aerobic exercises like walking, cycling, and jogging. Exercise helps control weight, a major contributor to insulin resistance, and enhances insulin sensitivity.

Prioritize Weight Management

Elevating body weight by just 5-10% can lead to a notable increase in insulin sensitivity. Prioritize sustained, long-term weight loss with exercise and a balanced diet.

Stress Management Techniques

Insulin resistance may deteriorate with ongoing stress. To control cortisol levels, engage in stress-reduction practices like yoga, meditation, deep breathing, or mindfulness.

Quality Sleep

Aim for 7-9 hours of quality sleep nightly. A consistent sleep schedule and a relaxing bedtime routine can significantly improve sleep quality.

By implementing these strategies, effective management of insulin resistance, and proper optimization of the body metabolism can be achieved.

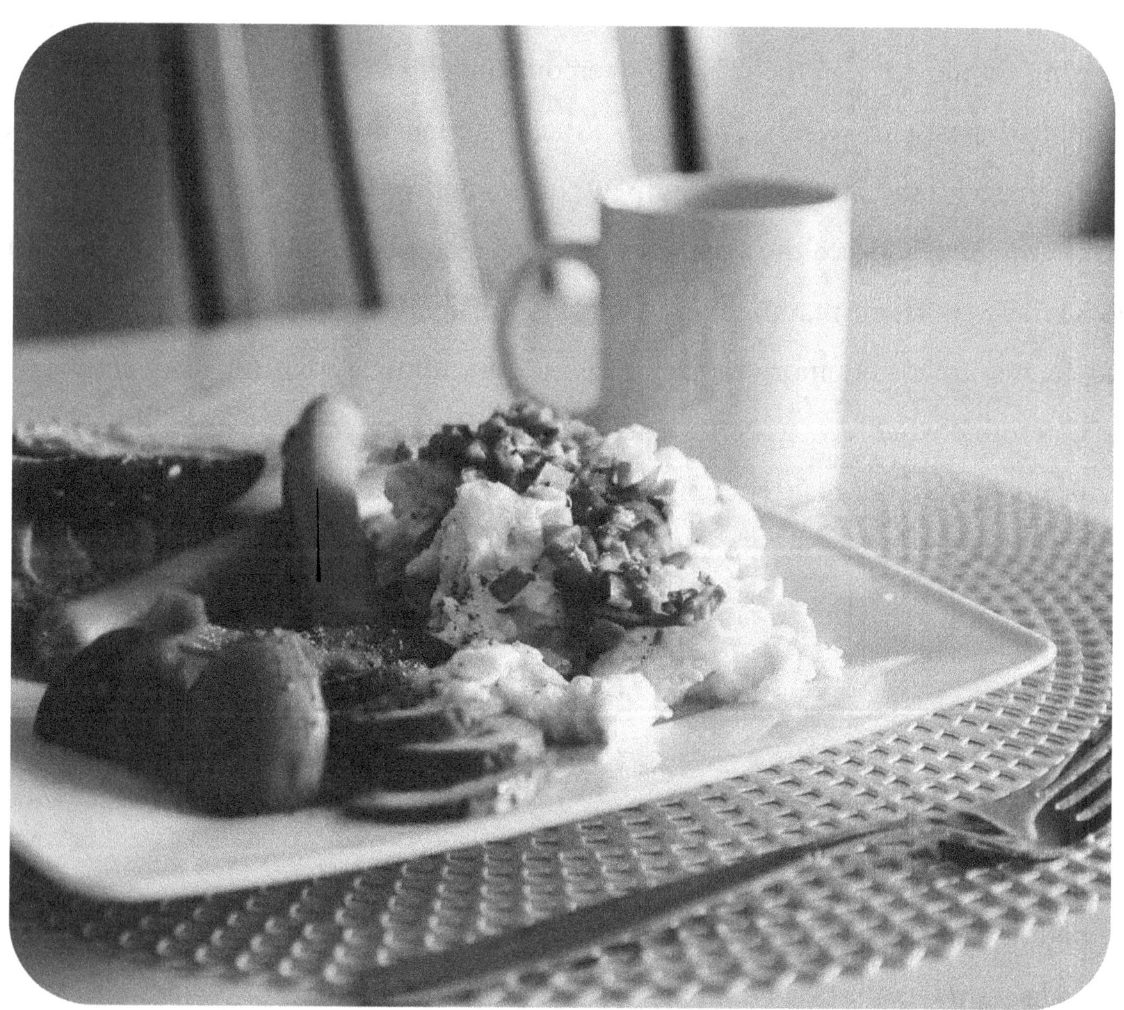

Chapter 3 - Endomorph Diet Explained

Tailoring your diet to your body type is key to optimizing your metabolism and hitting your health goals. For endomorphs, who naturally store fat more easily and have a slower metabolism, a strategic approach to nutrition is essential. The goal is to promote fat loss while maintaining muscle mass through a balanced diet. Here's how to customize your diet for optimal weight loss and overall health:

Key Principles:

Prioritize Nutrient-Dense Foods: Give priority to whole, unprocessed meals that are low in empty calories yet high in nutrients. These meals provide you with the vital vitamins and minerals your body needs while also helping you feel full and content.

Control Your Carbohydrate Intake: Because endomorphs are often more sensitive to carbs, they may store fat more quickly. Choose complex carbohydrates that have a low glycemic index, such as vegetables, legumes, and whole grains, since they will assist in regulating blood sugar levels and provide you with long-lasting energy.

Boost Protein Intake: Due to the thermic action of food, high-protein meals help you create and retain muscle mass while also increasing your metabolism. Incorporate plant-based proteins, fish, poultry, eggs, and other lean proteins into your meals.

Add Healthy Fats: Include healthy fats from foods like olive oil, avocados, nuts, and seeds. These fats keep you full and promote general wellness.

Regular, Balanced Meals: Eating smaller, more frequent well-balanced meals throughout the day will help control blood sugar levels and curb overindulgence.

Endomorph-Friendly Food Choices

Proteins:

- Lean meats (chicken, turkey, lean beef)
- Fish and seafood

- Eggs and egg whites
- Plant-based proteins (tofu, tempeh, legumes)
- Low-fat dairy products (Greek yogurt, cottage cheese)

Carbohydrates:

- Vegetables (leafy greens, cruciferous vegetables, peppers)
- Whole grains (quinoa, brown rice, oatmeal)
- Fruits (berries, apples, pears in moderation)
- Legumes (lentils, beans, chickpeas)

Fats:

- Avocados
- Nuts and seeds (almonds, chia seeds, flaxseeds)
- Healthy oils (olive oil, coconut oil)
- Fatty fish (salmon, mackerel, sardines)

Beverages:

- Water
- Herbal teas
- Coffee (in moderation)
- Avoid sugary drinks and limit alcohol consumption

Weight Loss Strategies for Endomorphs

Although losing weight can be difficult for endomorphs, it is undoubtedly possible with the appropriate strategy. Prioritize establishing a calorie deficit while making sure your body receives all the nutrients it requires for good health. So here's what you need to know:

Making a Deficit of Calories

- **Determine Your Basal Metabolic Rate (BMR):** Your daily caloric requirements can be ascertained by calculating your BMR. To determine this number, use online calculators or speak with a nutritionist.

- **Modify your caloric intake:** Try to eat fewer calories than your body requires to create a deficit, but avoid going below what is necessary to sustain your health or metabolism.

- **Portion Control:** To avoid overindulging, pay attention to the portion sizes. Portion management can be achieved by measuring food and using smaller plates.

Nutritional Timing:

- **Breakfast:** To boost your metabolism and keep you satisfied, start your day with a balanced meal high in protein and healthy fats.

- **Lunch and dinner:** Make sure your lunch and dinner have an appropriate ratio of protein, complex carbs, and healthy fats.

- **Snacks:** To sustain energy levels and stave off hunger, it is optimal to choose nutritious snacks like nuts, seeds, and veggies.

Foods to Limit or Avoid

On the endomorph diet, you should limit or stay away from the following foods as they can interfere with your progressive efforts to lose weights:

- **Refined Carbs:** White bread, pastries, and sugary cereals all lead to blood sugar spikes, and this in turn will promote fat storage which we are trying to curb.

- **Sugary Drinks and Foods:** Limit these empty calories that can lead to insulin resistance and hinder weight loss.

- **High-Fat Processed Foods:** Avoid fried foods, processed snacks, and fast food – they're loaded with calories and unhealthy fats.

- **Alcohol:** Limit alcohol consumption as it can slow metabolism and contribute to body fat.

Understanding Calories for Weight Management

Calories are units of energy in food. Our bodies require a specific amount to function properly. Here's how calories impact weight:

- **Calorie Balance:** When you consume the same amount of calories your body burns, you maintain your weight.

- **Calorie Surplus:** Eating more calories than you burn leads to weight gain as excess calories are stored as fat.

- **Calorie Deficit:** Eating fewer calories than your body burns results in weight loss as your body taps into fat reserves for energy.

Quality of Calories

Foods High in Nutrients: These offer vital nutrients without being overly caloric. Lean proteins, whole grains, and vegetables are a few examples.

Empty Calories: Foods poor in nutrition but heavy in sugar and bad fats are known as empty calories. Confectionery, soda, and junk food are a few examples.

Calorie Tracking for Weight Loss Success

Monitoring your calorie intake is crucial for the endomorph body type. Here are some methods to track your calories effectively:

- **Food Diaries:** Keeping a journal of your meals promotes accountability and awareness.

- **Calorie Tracking Apps:** Use apps like Lose It! or MyFitnessPal to easily log your food and monitor calorie intake.

- **Portion Control Techniques:** Follow serving sizes on food labels, utilize measuring cups and food scales for accurate portioning.

Tips for Effective Calorie Tracking:

- **Be Honest and Precise:** Record all your food and beverages consumed, no matter how small.

- **Make it a Habit:** Tracking your food intake should become a regular part of your routine.

- **Analyze and Adjust:** Regularly review your food journal to identify trends and make adjustments to stay within your calorie goals.

- **Make Use of Pre-Tracked Meal Plans:** There are numerous resources that provide recipes with pre-calculated calories and macros, such as Nutra check and MyFitness Pal. Make use of these to improve the accuracy and ease of tracking.

- **Track It If It's Packaged:** The barcode scanner found in most monitoring apps makes it simple to log packaged items. Track it if it has a barcode!

Chapter 4 - Nutrition for Endomorphs

Macronutrients for Endomorphs

For endomorphs aiming to maximize their nutrition and reach their health objectives, knowing macronutrients and their function in their diet is essential. This chapter will walk you through the suggested daily values, how to modify your macronutrient ratios, and useful advice for achieving your macronutrient objectives.

Macronutrients, which are fats, proteins, and carbs, are those nutrients your body needs in greater quantities, and each one has a different effect on your health and wellbeing.

Proteins: Each day, try to get 30–40% of your calories from protein. For the body to develop, repair, and maintain a healthy metabolism, protein is necessary. Lean meats, seafood, eggs, dairy products, legumes, and plant-based proteins are examples of sources.

Carbohydrates: Try to receive 25–30% of your daily energy from carbohydrates, with an emphasis on complex, low-GI carbohydrates. These include foods that balance blood sugar levels and offer prolonged energy, such as whole grains, veggies, and legumes.

Fats: Set aside 25–30% of your daily caloric intake for good fats. These are essential for brain function, hormone synthesis, and maintaining your feeling of fullness. Avocados, almonds, seeds, olive oil, and fatty seafood are excellent sources.

Although the aforementioned percentages are a useful place to start, it's crucial to modify these ratios in accordance with your unique requirements, activity levels, reactions, and particular health objectives.

Guidelines for Meeting Your Macronutrient Goals

Sticking to your daily macronutrient (macro) goals as an endomorph body type can feel tricky, but by adhering to the following strategies, one can leverage macros to support their metabolism, boost fitness efforts, and reach ideal health and weight management goals.

Plan Your Meals: Outline your meals and snacks in advance to ensure they meet your macro goals. You can simply track your meals and macros using apps like MyFitnessPal.

Balanced Plates: Make sure each meal includes a source of protein, good fat, and complex carbohydrates. Consider quinoa, avocado, and grilled chicken for a dish that is well-balanced.

Snacking wisely: Choose nibbles that complement your macros. Carrot sticks with hummus give a healthy carb and fat combination, while Greek yogurt with almonds provides both protein and excellent fats.

Protein Powders (Optional): If you feel that eating only plants can't help you reach your protein objectives, think about taking protein supplements like whey or plant-based powders. Use them as a post-workout snack, or add them to smoothies or porridge.

Healthy Cooking Techniques: Use little to no oil when you grill, bake, steam, or sauté food to maintain its nutritional value and flavor. Steer clear of deep-frying and extra harmful fats.

Staying Hydrated Is Essential: Getting adequate water is critical for good health because it aids in digestion and vitamin absorption. If you're an active person, try to get eight glasses or more each day.

Adapt and Adjust: Consistently assess your development and make necessary modifications. Pay attention to your body and adjust the macro ratios according to your energy levels and outcomes.

Micronutrient Needs for Endomorphs

While the focus is frequently on macronutrients, micronutrients are also pivotal for overall health and well-being. Micronutrients, including vitamins and minerals, play vital roles in maintaining health and supporting metabolism. While the specific requirements may vary, certain micronutrients are crucial for endomorphs. **Vitamin D**, frequently associated with bone health, also plays a part in cell growth modulation and vulnerable function. Some exploration suggests that adequate vitamin D levels may support weight management and metabolic health. **Magnesium**, a mineral, is involved in over 300 enzymatic responses in the body, including food metabolism and the conflation of adipose acids and proteins. Magnesium can help ameliorate metabolic profiles and has been associated with a reduced threat to metabolic patterns. Last but not least, **Iron** is essential for numerous metabolic processes and functions, including oxygen transport. Low iron levels can have an impact on metabolism and energy.

Supplements for the Endomorph Diet

Sustaining weight loss over the long run is a complex task, especially for endomorphs, whose natural tendency is to store fat. A mix of food adjustments, consistent exercise, and behavioral adjustments is required to achieve long-term weight loss. Supplements can help with these efforts, but they should be taken sparingly and as an addition to a healthy diet and regular exercise.

Why Supplemental Fiber Is Important

Because fiber supplements can aid digestion, control blood sugar, and increase satiety, they are especially helpful for endomorphs. Reducing calorie intake is linked to increasing dietary fiber consumption, which is important for managing weight. Fiber supplements, such as PolyGlycopleX (PGX), have demonstrated potential for supporting weight reduction through the facilitation of satiety, which lowers total caloric intake.

Components of Fiber Supplements for Weight Loss

Ingredients in effective fiber supplements are usually well-known for their advantageous physiological benefits. Important components of weight-loss fiber supplements include:

Glucomannan: This very viscous fiber, which is derived from the konjac root, swells in the stomach to increase fullness and decrease hunger.

Psyllium husk: This soluble fiber promotes healthy digestion and may have a lowering effect on cholesterol.

Inulin: A prebiotic fiber called inulin promotes gut health by feeding good microorganisms.

PGX, or PolyGlycopleX: PGX, a unique combination of sodium alginate, xanthan gum, and konjac glucomannan, is well-known for its high viscosity and capacity to solidify into a gel-like material in the stomach, improving satiety and regulating blood sugar levels.

The Benefits and Drawbacks of Fiber Supplements

Including fiber supplements in an endomorph's diet can have both benefits and drawbacks. On the positive side, fiber supplements increase satiety, helping you feel fuller for longer and reducing the likelihood of overeating. They also promote digestive health by aiding regular bowel movements and improving overall digestive function. Additionally, soluble fibers like PGX can help regulate blood sugar by slowing glucose absorption, preventing spikes. Fiber supplements can also aid in weight management by promoting fullness and reducing appetite, leading to a decrease in overall calorie intake. However, there are potential drawbacks. Rapidly increasing fiber intake can cause digestive discomfort such as bloating, gas, and abdominal pain. High fiber intake might interfere with the absorption of certain nutrients and medications. Moreover, relying solely on supplements for fiber can lead to neglecting whole food sources, which provide a wider range of nutrients essential for overall health.

Other Weight Loss Supplements for Endomorphs

When it comes to weight loss for endomorphs, certain supplements can potentially aid in the process. Now while these supplements can support weight loss efforts, they are not standalone solutions. Sustainable weight management relies on a balanced diet, regular exercise, and a healthy lifestyle. Always consult with a healthcare provider before starting any new supplement regimen.

Here's a breakdown of some popular options

Green coffee extracts

The green coffee extract, which is made out of unroasted coffee beans, contains chlogenic acids. These decrease blood sugar and insulin surges, leading to weight loss. However, some studies on its effectiveness have been conflicting.

HMB (Beta-Hydroxy Beta-Methylbutyrate)

Leucine is a very important amino acid, and its metabolite HMB slows down muscle breakdown and promotes muscle growth. While this may help retain weight during calorie deficits by sustaining lean body mass, more research needs to be done about these benefits.

Chromium Picolinate

Chromium picolinate is an essential mineral for both fat metabolism, carbohydrate metabolism, and even blood sugar control. Evidence indicating that it can aid in weight reduction by reducing appetite and food intake has not yet been provided by some trials.

Coleus Forskohlii

Forskolin, an extract from the root of India's indigenous Coleus forskohlii plant, has been used in medicine for a long time. Forskolin is believed to increase the activity of an enzyme that aids fat metabolism and breakdown. Despite its ancient use, there are mixed scientific findings concerning its effectiveness as a weight-loss aid.

Garcinia Cambogia

Garcinia cambogia is a tropical fruit known for its high hydroxycitric acid (HCA) content, which is believed to increase fat oxidation and suppress appetite. Several studies reveal that the program is beneficial for weight reduction, while others state that there are no notable effects.

Cayenne Pepper Extract

The cayenne pepper extract from Capsicum species has a hot taste, making it useful as a thermogenic. Consequently, capsaicin has been said to boost metabolism and reduce hunger, thereby lowering calorie intake and promoting weight loss. Nevertheless, different users may find it differently effective.

Caffeine Anhydrous

Caffeine anhydrous, a concentrated form of this stimulant, is typically found in dietary supplements used for athletic performance enhancement and weight loss. It can enhance lipolysis, focus, and metabolic rate. Effects of caffeine vary from person to person; excessive amounts might cause such symptoms as nervousness or sleeping difficulties.

Black pepper extract

Because piperine is present in black pepper extracts, it can aid in the absorption of other nutrients while also improving the efficiency of other supplements. Moreover, some research indicates that piperine could quicken metabolic processes leading to fat breakdown.

Chapter 5 - Endomorph Diet Recipes

Despite the fact that it may sound strange, you do not have to sacrifice flavor or variety when eating for your endomorph body type. There is a lot of fun and satisfaction in adopting a diet that meets the unique metabolic requirements of an endomorph. Eating foods that are nutrient dense, making sure macronutrients are balanced, emphasizing low-glycemic carbohydrates, and providing enough amounts of healthy fats and lean protein helps with weight management, health, and satiety. You will come across different delicious choices that will help endomorphs live well in this assortment of recipes. These meals have been crafted to fit into your day-to-day routines; hence, they can be eaten without disruption, from a hearty breakfast meant to kickstart your metabolism to fulfilling lunches and dinner meals in order to keep energy levels stable. In addition, there are also healthy snacks as well as desserts, ensuring that you don't compromise on your health goals while enjoying your food. Each recipe has taken into account the fact that the endomorph stores fat easily and takes longer than other body types to metabolize food. To manage insulin levels, promote fullness, and maintain muscles, these foods contain high fiber content, with the inclusion of lean protein on top of good fats. Furthermore, they do not contain any refined sugars or simple carbohydrates, which cause blood sugar spikes and fat storage.

So if you're looking for quick and easy meals or more classy dishes for special occasions, these endomorph-friendly recipes offer something for everyone. Enjoy the process of nourishing your body with foods that are both delicious and beneficial for your unique body. Embrace the journey towards a healthier, more balanced lifestyle with these tailored culinary creations.

Breakfast Recipes

Oatmeal with Peanut Butter & Banana

Preparation Time:

5 minutes

Cooking Time:

5 minutes

Number of Servings:

1

Ingredients:

- **1/2 cup rolled oats**
- **1 cup water or milk (for creamier texture)**
- **1 tablespoon peanut butter (natural, no added sugar)**
- **1 small banana, sliced**
- **1 teaspoon honey (optional)**
- **Pinch of salt**
- **Cinnamon (optional, for topping)**

Estimated Nutritional Information (Per Serving):

- **Calories: 310 kcal**
- **Protein: 11.5g**
- **Fat: 12g**
- **Carbohydrates: 38g**

Instructions:

1. In a small saucepan, bring some water or milk to a simmer.
2. Add a touch of salt and the rolled oats. Reduce the heat slightly and simmer, stirring occasionally, for five minutes.
3. Remove the saucepan from the heat once the oats have cooked and absorbed all of the liquid.
4. Add enough peanut butter to the mixture to coat everything evenly.
5. Scoop the oatmeal into a bowl and top it with sliced banana. If you want some sweetness, you may optionally sprinkle in some honey.
6. Add a little bit of cinnamon for the final touch.

Scrambled Eggs with Spinach and Tomato

Preparation Time:

5 minutes

Cooking Time:

5 minutes

Number of Servings:

1

Estimated Nutritional Information (Per Serving):

- **Calories: 200 kcal**
- **Protein: 14g**
- **Fat: 13g**
- **Carbohydrates: 5g**

Ingredients:

- **1/2 cup fresh spinach, chopped**
- **1 tablespoon milk or water**
- **1 teaspoon olive oil**
- **2 large eggs**
- **1/4 cup cherry tomatoes, halved**
- **Salt and pepper to taste**
- **Optional: 1 tablespoon grated cheese (like Parmesan or feta)**

Instructions:

1. In a small bowl, crack the eggs and whisk them with a little milk or water until smooth. For taste, don't forget to add a dash of salt and pepper!
2. In a nonstick pan, warm up some olive oil over medium heat.
3. Add the cherry tomatoes and simmer for one or two minutes, or until they begin to soften.
4. Cook the spinach for approximately a minute, or just until it wilts.
5. The major event is about to happen! Using a spatula, carefully whisk the egg mixture after pouring it into the pan. Continue cooking the eggs until they are set and attractively scrambled.
6. Before serving, sprinkle with a little grated cheese and allow it to melt a little. This makes a great dish.

Protein Pancakes

Preparation Time:

5 minutes

Cooking Time:

10 minutes

Number of Servings:

4

Estimated Nutritional Information (Per Serving):

- **Calories: 361 kcal**
- **Protein: 45.5g**
- **Fat: 11g**
- **Carbohydrates: 12.2g**

Ingredients:

- **2 Eggs**
- **½ cup Greek Yogurt**
- **⅓ cup Protein Powder**
- **½ tsp Cinnamon (optional)**
- **1-2 tbsp Oat Flour (optional, for thickening)**

Instructions:

1. Whisk eggs and yogurt in a bowl. Add protein powder and mix until smooth. Let batter thicken for 5 minutes.
2. Heat a greased griddle over medium heat.
3. Adjust batter consistency if needed (thicker = more protein powder, thinner = splash of milk).
4. Cook ¼ cup batter per pancake for 2-3 minutes per side, or until golden brown.
5. Serve with your favorite toppings!

Greek Yogurt Berry Parfait

Preparation Time:

5 minutes

Cooking Time:

None

Number of Servings:

1

Estimated Nutritional Information (Per Serving):

- **Calories: 251 kcal**
- **Protein: 22g**
- **Fat: 5g**
- **Carbohydrates: 29g**

Ingredients:

- **1 cup Greek yogurt (plain, non-fat)**
- **1 tablespoon maple syrup (optional)**
- **2 tablespoons granola (preferably low-sugar)**
- **1/2 cup mixed berries (blueberries, strawberries, raspberries)**
- **1 tablespoon chia seeds**

Instructions:

1. Half of the Greek yogurt should be layered in a glass or dish.
2. Spread some mixed berries over the yogurt.
3. Over the berries, spread the remaining Greek yogurt.
4. If desired, drizzle with maple syrup.
5. For added crunch and nutrients, sprinkle granola and chia seeds over top.
6. Serve immediately and enjoy!

Easy Blueberry Biscuits

Preparation Time:

15 minutes

Cooking Time:

24 minutes

Number of Servings:

6 -8 biscuits

Estimated Nutritional Information (Per Biscuit):

- **Calories: 257 kcal**
- **Protein: 6g**
- **Fat: 11g**
- **Carbohydrates: 29g**

Ingredients:

- **2 cups flour**
- **⅓ cup sugar**
- **1 tbsp baking powder**
- **½ tsp salt**
- **8 tbsp cold butter, cubed**
- **1 cup blueberries**
- **½ cup milk (add gradually)**

Instructions:

1. Line your baking pan with parchment paper.
2. In a bowl, whisk flour, sugar, baking powder, and salt. Cut in butter with a pastry cutter or fingers until crumbly.
3. Gently fold in blueberries and enough milk to form a dough.
4. Pat dough on a floured surface to a ¾-inch rectangle.
5. Use a 3-inch biscuit cutter to cut dough and arrange in pan, touching sides.
6. Refrigerate for 30 minutes and while they chill preheat oven to 425°F (220°C).
7. Bake 18-23 minutes or until golden brown.

Greek Yogurt Paired with Granola & Honey

Preparation Time:

5 minutes

Cooking Time:

None

Number of Servings:

1

Estimated Nutritional Information (Per Serving):

- **Calories: 264 kcal**
- **Protein: 18g**
- **Fat: 5g**
- **Carbohydrates: 38g**

Ingredients:

- **1 cup Greek yogurt (plain, non-fat)**
- **1/4 cup granola (preferably low-sugar)**
- **1 tablespoon honey**
- **1/4 teaspoon cinnamon (optional)**

Instructions:

1. Spoon the Greek yogurt into a bowl.
2. Top with granola.
3. Drizzle honey over the granola and yogurt.
4. Sprinkle with cinnamon if desired.
5. Serve immediately and enjoy!

Mashed Avocado and Salmon Bagel

Preparation Time:

10 minutes

Cooking Time:

None

Number of Servings:

1

Ingredients:

- **2 ounces smoked salmon**
- **1 tablespoon cream cheese (optional)**
- **1 tablespoon capers**
- **1 whole grain bagel, halved and toasted**
- **1/2 ripe avocado, mashed**
- **1/4 red onion, thinly sliced**
- **Fresh dill, for garnish**
- **Lemon wedge, for garnish**
- **2 tbsp sliced cucumbers**
- **Salt and pepper to taste**

Estimated Nutritional Information (Per Serving):

- **Calories: 379 kcal**
- **Protein: 20g**
- **Fat: 16g**
- **Carbohydrates: 36g**

Instructions:

1. Evenly divide the mashed avocado between the two toasted bagel halves.
2. Arrange the avocado and smoked salmon on top of it.
3. If you'd like, garnish with a dab of cream cheese.
4. Arrange the slices of red onion over the salmon and scatter with the capers.
5. Add a squeeze of lemon juice, fresh dill, and a piece of cucumber as garnish.
6. Add pepper and salt according to taste.
7. Serve right away, and savor!

Scrambled Eggs with Mushrooms

Preparation Time:

5 minutes

Cooking Time:

10 minutes

Number of Servings:

1

Ingredients:

- **1 teaspoon olive oil**
- **1/2 cup mushrooms, sliced**
- **1 small onion, finely chopped**
- **2 large eggs**
- **1/4 cup milk or water**
- **Salt and pepper to taste**
- **Fresh parsley, chopped (optional, for garnish)**

Estimated Nutritional Information (Per Serving):

- **Calories: 210 kcal**
- **Protein: 14g**
- **Fat: 15g**
- **Carbohydrates: 6g**

Instructions:

1. Beat the eggs with the milk or water in a small bowl until thoroughly combined. Add a dash of pepper and salt for seasoning.
2. In a nonstick skillet, warm the olive oil over medium heat.
3. Cook the chopped onions for 2 to 3 minutes, or until they become tender.
4. When the mushrooms are soft and the liquid has evaporated, add them and simmer for 4 to 5 minutes.
5. Transfer the egg mixture into the skillet and use a spatula to gently swirl until the eggs are cooked through and have a soft scrambled texture.
6. If preferred, top with fresh parsley after transferring to a platter.
7. Enjoy your meal

Tomato & Spinach Scrambled Eggs

Preparation Time:

10 minutes

Cooking Time:

None

Number of Servings:

1

Ingredients:

- **1/2 cup fresh spinach, chopped**
- **1 tablespoon milk or water**
- **1 teaspoon olive oil**
- **2 large eggs**
- **1/4 cup cherry tomatoes, halved**
- **1 tablespoon grated cheese (like Parmesan or feta)**
- **Salt and pepper to taste**

Estimated Nutritional Information (Per Serving):

- **Calories: 200 kcal**
- **Protein: 14g**
- **Fat: 14g**
- **Carbohydrates: 5g**

Instructions:

1. In a little dish, thoroughly beat the eggs with the milk or water. Grind in some salt and pepper.
2. Warm the olive oil in an ovenproof pan over medium heat.
3. Stirring occasionally, cook the cherry tomatoes until they start to soften, one to two minutes.
4. Cook the spinach, stirring, until it wilts, approximately a minute.
5. Spoon the egg mixture into the skillet, swirling with a spatula, and heat until the eggs are soft scrambled.
6. Before serving, throw grated cheese over and leave it to melt a little.

Oatmeal Pancakes with Greek Yogurt

Preparation Time:

5 minutes

Cooking Time:

15 minutes

Number of Servings:

8-10 pancakes

Ingredients:

- **2 tablespoons granulated sugar (or coconut sugar)**
- **1 cup vanilla Greek yogurt**
- **1 teaspoon vanilla extract**
- **2 eggs, lightly beaten**
- **1 teaspoon baking powder**
- **½ teaspoon baking soda**
- **½ teaspoon fine sea salt**
- **½ teaspoon cinnamon**
- **1 cup oat flour (or wheat flour)**
- **¼ cup all-purpose flour (or gluten-free all-purpose flour)**
- **1-2 tablespoons milk (regular, almond, or coconut), if needed.**
- **Salted butter or coconut oil (for greasing the skillet)**

Estimated Nutritional Information (Per Serving):

- **Calories: 65.9 kcal**
- **Carbohydrates: 12g**
- **Protein: 8g**
- **Fat: 1.9g**

Instructions:

1. Preheat an electric griddle to 350 degrees.
2. In a large bowl, beat together the eggs, vanilla, and Greek yogurt until creamy.
3. In a separate dish, stir together the sugar, cinnamon, baking powder, baking soda, all-purpose flour, and oat flour.
4. Stir thoroughly to combine the dry ingredients with the wet ones. If the batter is too thick to reach the desired consistency, add one tablespoon of milk at a time.
5. Melt the coconut oil or butter on the griddle or pan.
6. Spoon pancake batter onto ½ cup portions on the heated, greased surface.
7. Simmer the mixture for two to four minutes, stirring now and again, or until the edges firm and bubble.
8. After they get golden brown, grill them for a further two to four minutes on the other side.

Whole Grain Breakfast Pancakes

Preparation Time:

10 minutes

Cooking Time:

10 minutes

Number of Servings:

2 pancakes

Ingredients:

- **1 cup buttermilk**
- **1 cup whole wheat flour**
- **1 tablespoon sugar**
- **1 teaspoon baking powder**
- **2 tablespoons melted butter or olive oil**
- **1 teaspoon vanilla extract**
- **1/2 teaspoon baking soda**
- **1/4 teaspoon salt**
- **1 large egg**
- **Olive oil or cooking spray (for the pan)**

Estimated Nutritional Information (Per Serving):

- **Calories: 181 kcal**
- **Protein: 8g**
- **Fat: 8g**
- **Carbohydrates: 26g**

Instructions:

1. Mix in a large bowl the salt, baking soda, baking powder, sugar, and whole wheat flour.
2. Combine the egg, buttermilk, vanilla essence, and olive oil or melted butter in another basin.
3. Stirring just enough, add the wet components to the dry ones. The batter should be a touch lumpy, not overmixed.
4. Turn on a medium-heat nonstick pan or griddle and brush with cooking spray or olive oil.
5. Pour each pancake onto the skillet using about 1/4 cup batter.
6. Two to three minutes later, the pancake should start to bubble on top. Cook, flipping once again, for a further one to two minutes, or until well-cooked and golden.
7. Continue with the leftover batter.

Veggie & Cheese Omelette

Preparation Time:

10 minutes

Cooking Time:

30 minutes

Number of Servings:

4

Ingredients:

- **40g butter**
- **300ml thickened cream**
- **4 tomatoes, halved**
- **1 red capsicum pepper (deseeded, diced)**
- **600g rye bread, sliced**
- **1 pinch pepper & salt**
- **8 eggs**
- **200g cup mushrooms**
- **425g tin green asparagus (diced)**
- **2 tbs olive oil**
- **1 cup tasty cheese (shredded)**

Estimated Nutritional Information (Per Serving):

- **Calories: 181 kcal**
- **Protein: 22g**
- **Fat: 12g**
- **Carbohydrates: 17g**

Instructions:

1. Warm the oven up to 200°C. Put baking paper on a tray.
2. Arrange the tomato on the paper. Pour in one tablespoon of olive oil and season with salt and pepper. Roast for about 20 minutes until soft.
3. Put the asparagus in a bowl that can withstand heat and pour boiling water over it. After a minute, thoroughly drain and put back into the bowl.
4. In a frying pan, heat the remaining oil over medium to high heat. Put in the mushrooms and simmer them for 5 minutes or until it's golden brown. add the capsicum and simmer for 3 minutes Spoon into a bowl and add the asparagus. Add seasoning and stir.
5. In a separate bowl, whisk together the eggs and cream. Melt 10g of butter in a small omelette pan over medium heat. Once the butter is sizzling, pour in a quarter of the egg mixture, swirling the pan to coat the bottom.
6. As the egg begins to set around the edges, use a spatula to gently drag the cooked egg towards the center of the pan. Once mostly set, sprinkle a quarter of the vegetable mixture and a quarter of the cheese on the half of the omelette furthest from the handle. Fold the other half over the filling.
7. Transfer the omelet to a platter for serving. Proceed in the same manner with the leftover cheese, egg mixture, vegetable filling, and butter. Add tomato and parsley to the top of each omelette. Accompany with rye bread.

Chapter 6 - Lunch Recipes

Grilled Chicken Salad

Preparation Time:

10 minutes

Cooking Time:

15 minutes

Number of Servings:

4

Ingredients:

Salad:

- 8 bowls assorted greens

Sliced vegetables:

- 1/2 cucumber
- 1/4 red onion (thinly sliced)
- 1 cup cherry tomatoes (halved)

Chicken Marinade:

- 2 tablespoons balsamic vinegar
- 1 tablespoon Dijon mustard
- 4 boneless chicken breasts (approx. 1 lb)
- 1 tablespoon olive oil
- 1 teaspoon garlic powder
- 1 teaspoon oregano
- Salt and pepper

Instructions

Grill the Chicken:

1. Heat your grill to medium-high.

2. In a bowl, mix olive oil, spices, and seasonings. Rub this marinade onto the chicken breasts.

3. Cook the chicken on the grill for 5 to 7 minutes on each side, until the internal temperature reaches a fully cooked state. Let it rest for 5 minutes, then slice or chop it into bite-sized pieces.

Assemble the Salad:

1. Toss together mixed greens, tomatoes, cucumber, and red onion in a large bowl.
2. To make a basic dressing, mix Dijon mustard and balsamic vinegar in a separate bowl.
3. To coat everything, drizzle the dressing over the salad and mix.
4. Finally, top your delicious creation with the grilled chicken pieces!

Estimated Nutrition Information (per serving)

- Calories: 300 kcal
- Protein: 35g
- Fat: 10g
- Carbs: 15g

Grilled Salmon and Asparagus

Preparation Time:

10 minutes

Cooking Time:

13 minutes

Number of Servings:

4

Ingredients

4 salmon fillets (around 6 oz each)

1 pound asparagus, trimmed

2 tablespoons olive oil

2 garlic cloves, minced

1 lemon, sliced

Salt and pepper to taste

Fresh dill or parsley (optional, for garnish)

Instructions

1. Get your grill nice and hot, cranking it to medium-high heat.
2. In a bowl, whip up a marinade by mixing olive oil, minced garlic, salt, and pepper.
3. Brush half of this flavorful mixture onto the salmon fillets. Don't forget the other half – toss your trimmed asparagus in it for extra taste!
4. Time to grill! Place the salmon on the grill, skin side down, for 6-7 minutes per side. You're looking for that perfectly cooked salmon: opaque and flakes easily with a fork.

5. Once the salmon's grilled, add the asparagus to the party. Cook for 8–10 minutes, turning them every now and then, until they're tender and have some nice char marks.

6. Plate your delicious creation: grilled salmon with asparagus. Top it off with lemon slices, parsley, or fresh dill for a beautiful and tasty finish (optional, but recommended!).

Estimated Nutrition Information (per serving)

- Calories: 289 kcal
- Protein: 29g
- Fat: 18g
- Carbohydrates: 5g

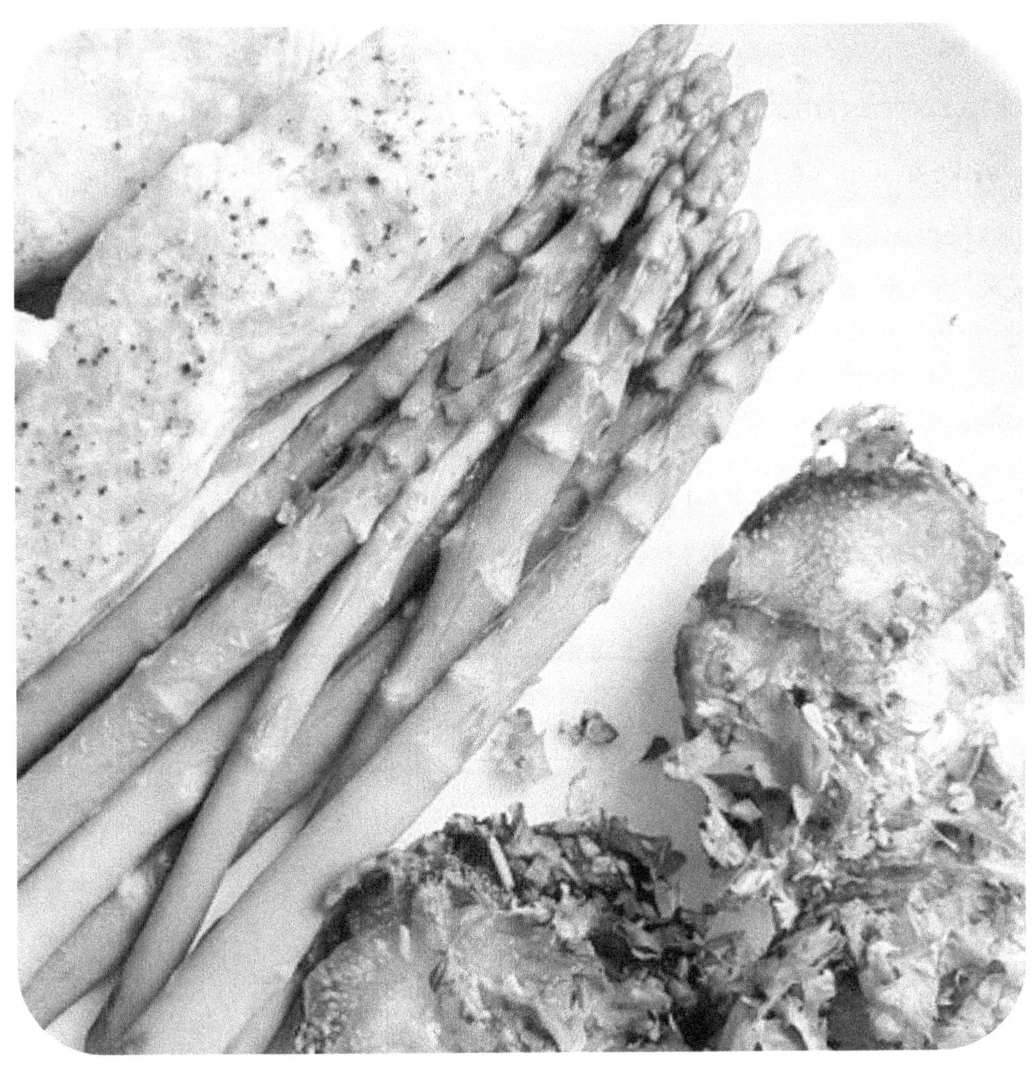

Mixed Greens & Avocado Chicken Salad

Preparation Time:

15 minutes

Cooking Time:

15 minutes

Number of Servings:

4

Ingredients

For the Chicken:

- 2 chicken breasts (around 8 oz each)
- 2 tbsp olive oil (for cooking)
- Salt and pepper to taste

For the Salad:

- 6 cups mixed salad greens
- 1 avocado, diced
- 1 cup cherry tomatoes, halved
- 1 cucumber, sliced
- 1/4 red onion, thinly sliced

For the Creamy Balsamic Dressing:

- 2 tbsp olive oil
- 1 tbsp balsamic vinegar
- 1 tsp Dijon mustard
- 1 garlic clove, minced
- Salt and pepper to taste

Instructions

1. First, toss in some salt and pepper to your chicken breasts.
2. In a skillet set over medium-high heat, add two teaspoons of olive oil. Add the chicken when it's heated, and cook it for seven to eight minutes on each side. Check the inside temperature, too; for safety, it should reach 165°F (74°C).
3. Slice up the cooked chicken after letting it rest for five minutes.
4. Measure out the olive oil, balsamic vinegar, Dijon mustard, minced garlic, salt, and pepper into a small bowl. You now have a lovely, thick balsamic dressing!
5. In a big bowl, add the red onion, cherry tomatoes, cucumber, cubed avocado, and mixed greens. This is your foundation for the salad.
6. Top it with the previously prepared sliced chicken.
7. After drizzling the creamy balsamic dressing on the salad, toss it carefully to bathe everything in taste.

Estimated Nutrition Information (per serving)

- Calories: 441 kcal
- Protein: 22g
- Fat: 29g
- Carbohydrates: 13g

Tip

For the perfect avocado, pick one with darker skin. Gently squeeze it in your palm (not with your fingers). If it yields a bit, it's ripe and ready to enjoy!

This dressing can be sweetened with honey, but if you're following a keto diet, skip it altogether.

Chickpea Salad Sandwich

Preparation Time:

15 minutes

Cooking Time:

0 minutes

Number of Servings:

4

Ingredients

For the Chickpea Salad:

- 1 can (15 oz) chickpeas, drained and rinsed
- 1 celery stalk, finely chopped
- 1 small red onion, finely chopped
- ¼ cup plain Greek yogurt
- 1 tbsp Dijon mustard
- 1 tbsp lemon juice
- Salt and pepper to taste

For the Sandwich Assembly:

- 2 slices whole grain bread
- 1 cup mixed greens (lettuce, spinach, arugula, etc.)
- 1 avocado, sliced

Instructions

1. Get a medium-sized bowl and use a fork to smash the chickpeas until they are nicely chunky.
2. Add all of the delicious things now, including the chopped celery, red onion, Greek yogurt, Dijon mustard, lemon juice, salt and pepper. Till everything is spread equally, swirl everything together.
3. Set out your pieces of whole-grain bread like a delectable runway.
4. On half of the slices—four—douse liberally with the chickpea salad.
5. Toppers time! Top with gorgeous slices of avocado and scatter over some mixed leaves.
6. Remember the other half of the bread! Set the remaining slices gently on top.
7. Slice the sandwiches in half and start eating straight away!

Estimated Nutrition Information (per serving)

- Calories: 287 kcal
- Protein: 15g
- Fat: 5g
- Carbohydrates: 35g

Tuna Salad Sandwich

Preparation Time:

15 minutes

Cooking Time:

0 minutes

Number of Servings:

6

Ingredients

1 teaspoon Dijon mustard

1 teaspoon lemon juice

1/4 teaspoon salt

1/4 teaspoon pepper

8 slices wheat bread

12 oz white flaked tuna in water, drained

1 stalk celery, finely diced

1 green onion, sliced

3/4 cup mayonnaise

2 dill pickle spears, finely chopped

Instructions

1. To prepare the tuna, make sure it is well-drained of any extra water.
2. In a small bowl, thoroughly mix the mayonnaise, Dijon mustard, lemon juice, chopped dill pickles, diced celery, sliced green onion, salt, and pepper.
3. Use the tuna salad as a salad topping, in sandwiches, or mixed into pasta salads.

Estimated Nutrition Information (per serving)

- Calories: 246 kcal
- Carbohydrates: 2g
- Protein: 12g
- Fat: 22g
-

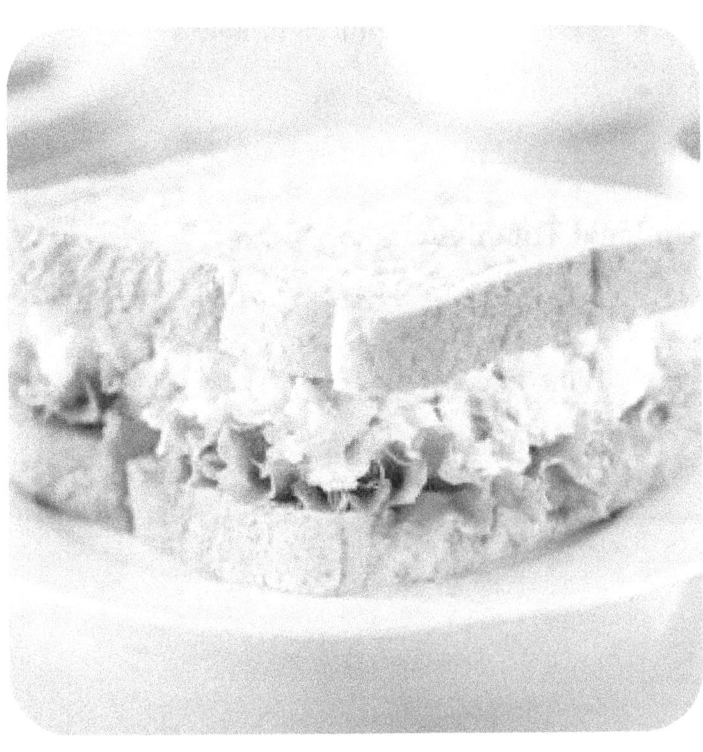

Black Bean & Sweet Potato Bowl

Preparation Time:

15 minutes

Cooking Time:

25 minutes

Number of Servings:

3

Ingredients

- 1 medium sweet potato, peeled and cubed (cooked)
- 1 cup cooked black beans
- 1 red bell pepper, diced
- 1 avocado, sliced
- 1 cup chopped spinach or kale
- 1 tablespoon olive oil
- Salt and pepper to taste

Optional Toppings:

- Salsa
- Lime juice
- Fresh cilantro

Instructions

1. Get your oven nice and hot, preheating it to 400°F (200°C).

2. Toss the cubed sweet potatoes with some olive oil, salt, and pepper to coat them in flavor.

3. Spread the seasoned sweet potatoes in a single layer on a baking sheet and roast them for 20-25 minutes, or until they're tender and cooked through.

4. While the sweet potatoes are roasting, you can prep the other ingredients. Get your black beans, diced red pepper, sliced avocado, and chopped spinach or kale ready.

5. In a large bowl, combine all these prepped ingredients.

6. Once the sweet potatoes are out of the oven, add them to the bowl with the other ingredients.

7. Drizzle with a bit more olive oil if you want some extra moisture, and season everything with salt and pepper to taste.

8. Now comes the fun part: toppings! If you want a flavor boost, add some salsa, a squeeze of fresh lime juice, or some chopped cilantro (or all three!).

Give everything a good mix and dig into your delicious and healthy Black Bean & Sweet Potato Bowl!

Estimated Nutrition Information (per serving)

- Calories: 276 kcal

- Protein: 9g

- Fat: 12g

- Carbohydrates: 31g

Turkey with Avocado Salad

Preparation Time:

10 minutes

Cooking Time:

0

Number of Servings:

4

Ingredients

- 4 cups cooked turkey breast, shredded into bite-sized pieces (about 2 inches)
- 1/2 cup diced red onion
- 1/2 cup roughly chopped cilantro
- 2 1/2 large ripe avocados, pitted (with the option to add more)
- 2 chopped jalapenos
- 2 limes, juiced (with extra for adjusting flavor)
- 2 diced celery stalks
- 1/2 tsp sea salt (with extra for adjusting flavor)
- 1/4 tsp black pepper (with extra for adjusting flavor)
- 1/4 tsp crushed red pepper (optional, for a spicy kick

Crunchy Toppings:

- 1/4 cup chopped pecans
- 1/4 cup sliced almonds
- 1/4 cup dried cranberries

Instructions

1. Prepare the vegetables: Chop the jalapenos, cilantro, and red onion.

2. Toss in the chopped pecans, chopped almonds, dried cranberries, chopped jalapenos, chopped red onion, chopped cilantro, and diced celery in a big bowl.

3. Smash the Avocado: Add the avocados to the bowl and bash them into the concoction with forks.

4. To season, add the crushed red pepper (if using), black pepper, lime juice, and sea salt. Combine them all thoroughly.

5. Taste and adjust: For more zest or creaminess, add extra lime juice or avocado.

6. Serve: If preferred, top the salad with more lime juice and serve straight away.

Estimated Nutrition Information (per serving)

- Calories: 368 kcal
- Protein: 43.6g
- Fat: 12g
- Carbohydrates: 11g

Tips

- Chop up and stir in a cooked egg for extra protein.
- Roasted turkey breast can be replaced with deli or ground turkey.
- If dairy is okay for you, shred some cheddar or Swiss cheese.

Chicken and Veggie Tacos

Preparation Time:

10 minutes

Cooking Time:

30 minutes

Number of Servings:

4

Ingredients

---

1 lb chicken thighs or breast

Marinade (mix these ingredients):

- 2 tbsp oil
- 2 tbsp low-sodium tamari (or soy sauce)
- 2 tbsp lime juice
- 1/2 tsp each of cumin, coriander, paprika, and oregano

Veggies:

- 2 peppers (any color, sliced)
- 3 large carrots (sliced)
- Seasoning (mix these ingredients):
    - 2 tbsp oil
    - 1/2 tsp each of paprika, cumin, coriander, and oregano
- Salt and pepper to taste

Jalapeno Sauce:

- 2 jalapenos (thinly sliced)

- 2 tbsp oil
- 1/4 cup low-sodium tamari (or soy sauce)
- 2 tbsp lime juice

Taco Fixings:

- Corn tortillas
- Sliced radishes
- Cilantro

Instructions

1. In a dish, toss together the chicken thighs and all the marinade ingredients; cover and refrigerate. While the chicken marinades, time to cut the vegetables!
2. In a large bowl, toss the sliced carrots and peppers with the oil and spices. Check that every surface is covered equally.
3. On a sprayed baking pan, spread the vegetables out, leaving room between them. Turn them halfway through the 15-minute high-heat broiling. They should still have a little sharp snap to them, but be softened and somewhat burned. When finished, remove them and set them aside.
4. Put the marinaded chicken thighs on the same baking sheet when the vegetables are done. Halfway through the ten minutes, you broil them and flip them. Take a thermometer reading inside; it should be 165°F.
5. In a small saucepan set over medium heat, whisk up the jalapeno sauce. Cook the sliced jalapenos, turning frequently, for five minutes until they soften.
6. To make your zesty sauce, turn off the heat and whisk in the tamari and lime juice.
7. Now, warm up your tortillas in an ungreased pan over medium heat, or even hold them over an open flame for a smoky touch.

8. Prepare your tacos! Stuff them with slices of jalapeño, roasted peppers, and carrots. Also, add the shredded chicken and the slicings of radish and fresh cilantro to round it out. Don't forget to provide those who want their food really hot some more jalapeño sauce on the side!

Estimated Nutrition Information (per serving)

- Calories: 381 kcal
- Protein: 28g
- Fat: 19g
- Carbohydrates: 17g

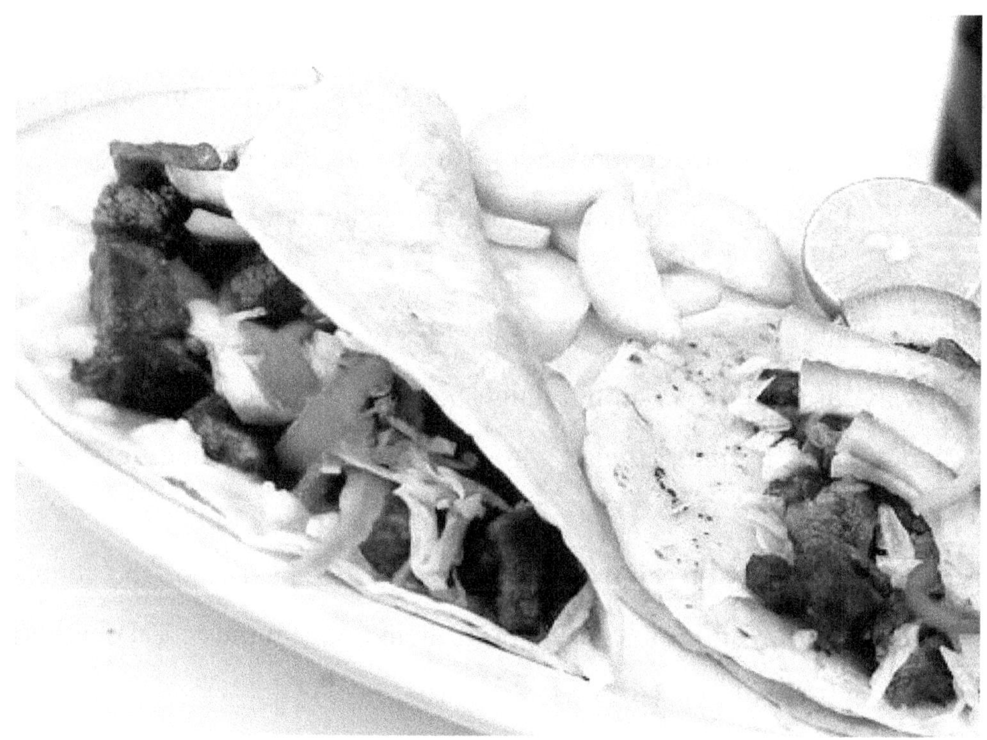

Grilled Zucchini and Quinoa Salad

Preparation Time:

20 minutes

Cooking Time:

25 minutes

Number of Servings:

6

Ingredients

- 1 cup quinoa
- 4 big, zucchini (lengthwise: quartered)
- 1/2 cup extra virgin olive oil
- 1 1/2 teaspoon sea salt (divided)
- 1 big clove of garlic
- 2 spring onions (parts light green and white)
- 1/2 cup of toasted almonds (plus extra for garnish)
- 1 1/2 coriander bunches
- 6 thinly sliced radishes, ends chopped
- 3 big limes' zest and juice (approximately 1/3 cup juice)
- 1/3 cup extra virgin olive oil
- 1/2 cup crumbled goat cheese (plus extra for decoration)

Instructions

Cooking the Quinoa:

1. Give it a good rinse till the water flows clear.
2. Boil some water in a pot and season with salt. Return the quinoa, rinsed, to a boil.
3. Simmer, covered, over low heat, until quinoa is fluffy and cooked, about 15 minutes. When finished, set it aside to cool.

Grilling the Zucchini

4. Preheat your grill pan well. Toss the zucchini in salt and olive oil.
5. About seven minutes later, the zucchini should be soft and have excellent char marks from being grilled over high heat, rotating once.
6. When they're done, move them to a chopping board and cut them into bite-sized pieces.

Directions for the Almond Coriander Pesto:

7. Blend the garlic, spring onions, almonds, most of the coriander, and lime juice. Blitz until silky.
8. Drizzle in olive oil little by little until the mixture takes on the consistency of pesto. If necessary, incorporate more spices and oil.

Making Your Salad

9. Stir some of the pesto into the cooked quinoa in a big bowl.
10. Add the remaining coriander, chopped fine, to the bowl.
11. Add the crumbled goat cheese, sliced radishes, and grilled zucchini—taste-test everything for salt and pepper.

Serving Up the Goodness: Arrange your mouthwatering dish and top with more goat cheese and toasted almonds for a last flourish!

Estimated Nutrition Information (per serving)

- Calories: 321 kcal
- Protein: 13g
- Fat: 13g
- Carbohydrates: 22g

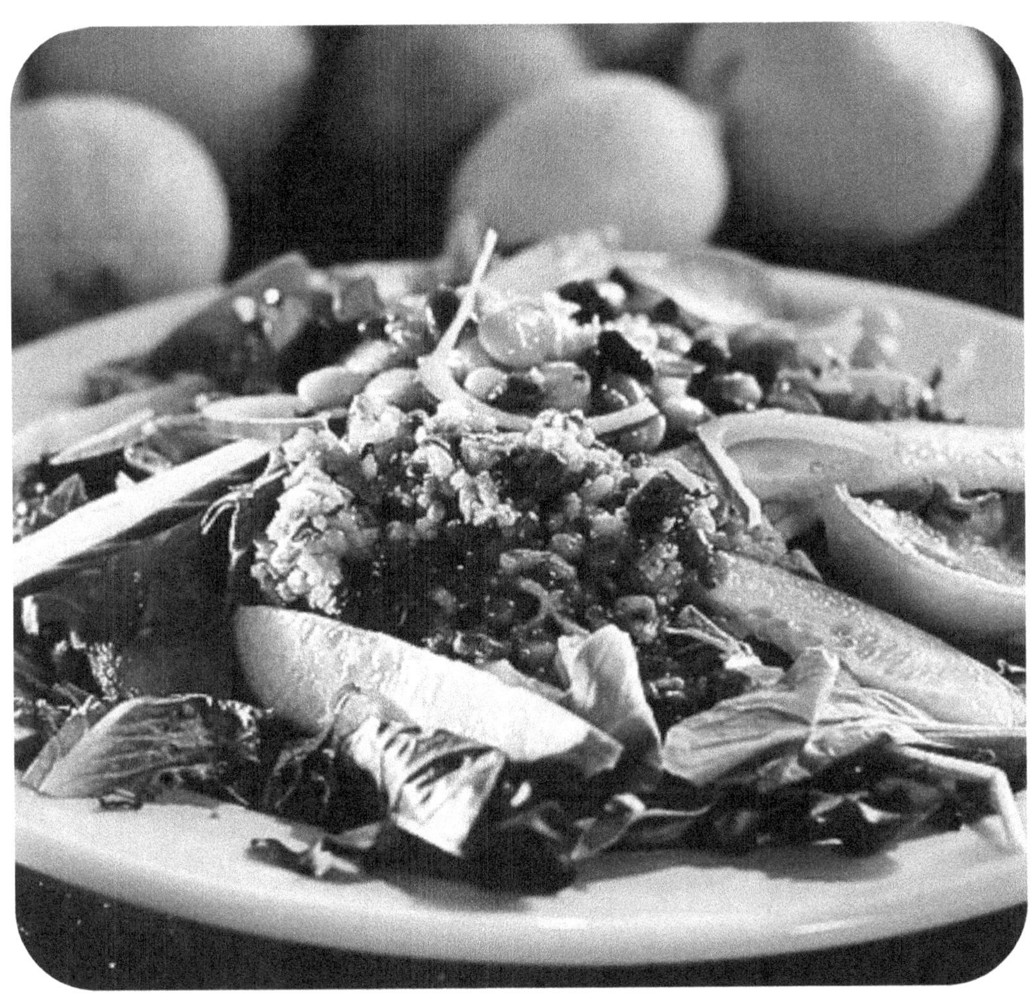

Grilled Chicken and Bean Salad

Preparation Time:

25 minutes

Refrigeration Time:

2 hours

Number of Servings:

4

Ingredients

Salad:

- 4 boneless, skinless chicken breast halves
- 1 can pinto beans, drained and rinsed
- 4 cups firmly packed gourmet salad greens
- 4 bacon slices, crisply cooked, drained, crumbled
- 1/4 cup chopped walnuts, toasted

Dressing:

- 1/4 cup maple syrup
- 2 tablespoons cider vinegar
- 1 teaspoon Dijon mustard
- 1/4 teaspoon salt
- 1/4 teaspoon pepper
- 1/4 cup vegetable oil

Instructions

Making the Dressing:

1. Grab a large bowl and whisk together all the dressing ingredients until everything's well combined.

2. Time to marinate the chicken! Pour out 1/4 cup of the dressing into a resealable plastic bag. Add the chicken breasts, seal the bag tightly, and shake it around to coat the chicken evenly. Pop the bag in the fridge for 2 hours to marinate. Keep the rest of the dressing aside for later.

Grilling Up the Chicken:

3. Heat your grill (gas or charcoal) to medium heat.

4. Grill the chicken for 10-12 minutes, flipping it once halfway through. You want the chicken to be cooked through (no pink in the center) and reach an internal temperature of 165°F. Let it cool slightly, then slice it crosswise.

Putting Together the Salad:

5. Toss all the remaining salad ingredients in the bowl with the leftover dressing you set aside earlier. Make sure everything is coated!

6. Divide the delicious salad mixture among 4 plates and top each plate with the sliced chicken breast.

Toasting the Walnuts (Optional):

7. If you want some toasted walnuts for an extra crunch, heat a small nonstick skillet over medium-low heat.

8. Add the walnuts and cook them for 2-3 minutes, stirring often, until they're lightly toasted. Be careful not to burn them! Take them off the heat right away.

9. Enjoy your meal.

Estimated Nutrition Information (per serving)

- Calories: 440 kcal
- Protein: 30g
- Fat: 20g
- Carbohydrates: 18g

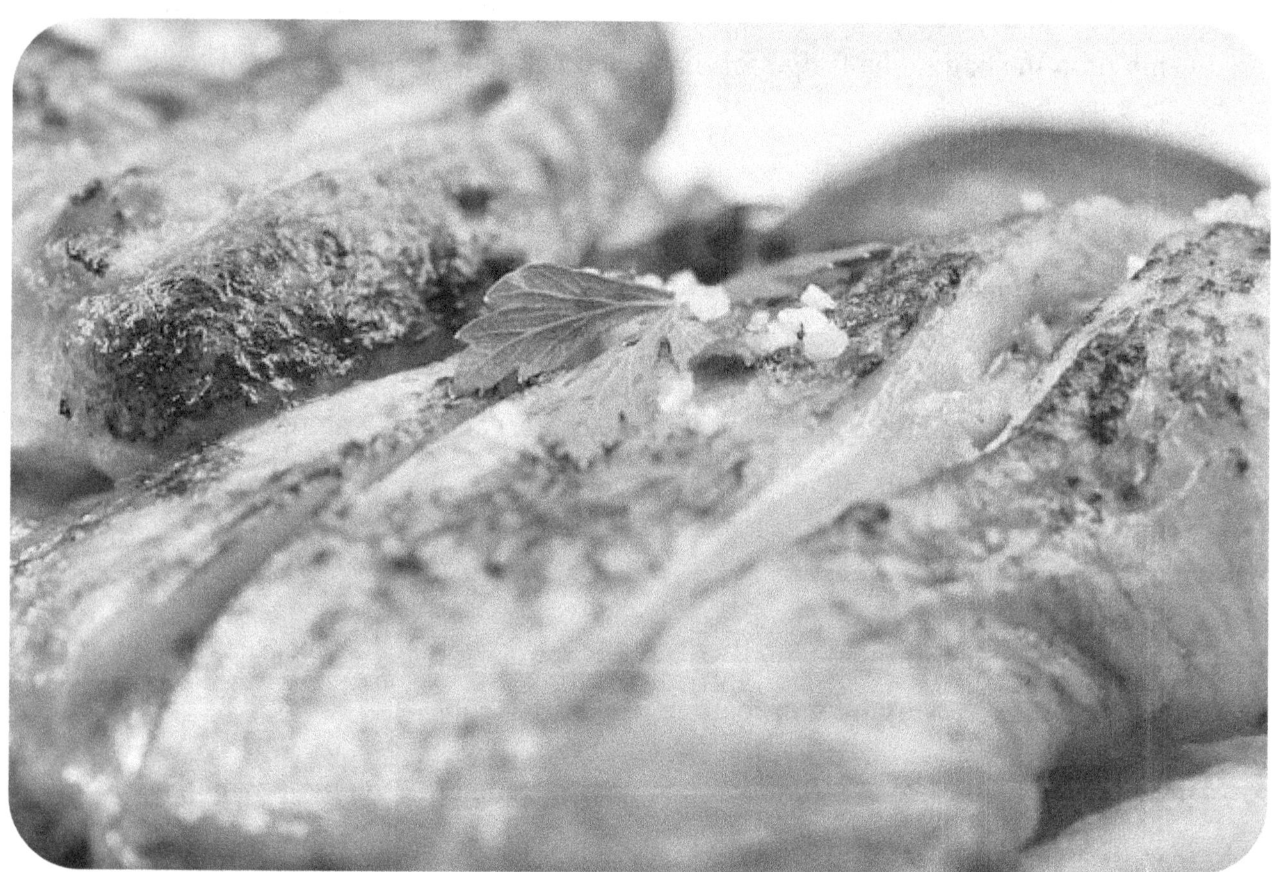

Vegetables and Roasted Pork Tenderloin

Preparation Time:

10 minutes

Refrigeration Time:

25 minutes

Number of Servings:

4

Ingredients

- 2 pounds pork tenderloin (1 or 1.5 pounds each)
- **For the Glaze:**
    - 1/4 cup honey
    - 3 garlic cloves, minced
    - 3 tablespoons coarsely ground mustard (deli mustard works too)
    - 3-4 sprigs of rosemary, finely chopped
    - 3 tablespoons white wine
    - 3 tablespoons extra-virgin olive oil
    - Salt and pepper to taste
- 1.5 pounds Yukon Gold potatoes, unpeeled and quartered
- 1 pound green beans, trimmed
- Pan spray or olive oil

Instructions

---

1. Turn the oven on high heat (450°F, 230°C).

2. First, you'll prepare the glaze by tossing the garlic, honey, mustard, wine, rosemary, salt, and pepper in a bowl with the olive oil.

3. Now pat the pork dry and then sprinkle it with pepper. Brush the pork thickly with the glaze.

4. Apply some olive oil or pan spray onto a baking sheet and give it a quick spritz. Line up the green beans along the middle, making room for the potatoes on either side. After seasoning with salt and pepper, put the potatoes, skin side down, in the pan.

5. Carefully place the glazed pork tenderloins on top of the green beans, ensuring that each pork does not touch. Apply the remaining glaze by brushing them one more time. Roast for 20-25 minutes, or until the pork achieves an internal temperature of 140°F (60°C).

6. Transfer the pork to a chopping board, tent with foil, and let it rest for 10 minutes while the veggies finish cooking.

7. Increase the oven temperature to 475°F (245°C) and roast the veggies for additional 5-10 minutes, or until soft and golden.

8. Serve: Transfer veggies to a plate. Slice the rested pork into ½-inch thick slices and lay over the veggies. Drizzle with any pan juices and enjoy!

Chapter 7 - Dinner Recipes

Grilled Shrimp and Veggie Skewers

Preparation Time:

5 minutes

Marinating Time:

2 hours

Cooking Time:

15 minutes

Number of Servings:

4

Ingredients

For the Shrimp (makes 4 skewers):

- 1 lb jumbo shrimp, peeled and deveined
- 1/2 cup plain non-fat Greek yogurt
- 1/4 cup lemon juice
- 1/2 tsp dried dill
- 1/2 tsp dried oregano
- 1/2 tsp kosher salt
- 2 garlic cloves, minced

For the Vegetables (makes 8 skewers):

- 1-pint cherry tomatoes
- 1 bunch asparagus, trimmed and cut into 1.5-2" pieces

- 1 red onion, chopped into large chunks
- 1 tbsp red wine vinegar
- 1 tsp olive oil
- 1/2 tsp kosher salt
- 1/4 tsp dried dill
- 1/4 tsp dried oregano
- 2 garlic cloves, minced

Instructions

For the shrimp:

1. Mix the Marinade: Whisk the Greek yogurt, lemon juice, minced garlic, dill, oregano, and kosher salt together in a bowl.
2. Add the shrimp to the marinade, cover, and chill for at least four hours.
3. Thread the shrimp onto metal or wooden skewers. If utilizing an outside barbecue, dunk wooden skewers in water before use.
4. The shrimp should be cooked thoroughly after being turned once on a grill pan or outside grill set over medium-high heat.

For the vegetables:

5. Gather the vegetables. Brush the veggies. After trimming the asparagus, cut it into 1.5 to 2" pieces. Finely chop the red onion.
6. Add the minced garlic, dill, oregano, kosher salt, and red wine vinegar to a small bowl to make the vinaigrette.
7. For variation, alternately thread the veggies onto metal or wooden skewers. For an outside barbecue, soak wooden skewers in water.

8. To marinate the vegetables, arrange the skewers on a plate and drizzle with the vinaigrette. When you're ready to cook, let them sit.

9. If using a grill pan, cover with a lid and turn the vegetables frequently throughout the approximately ten minutes of grilling. Before serving, drizzle the grilled skewers with whatever vinaigrette is left.

Estimated Nutrition Information (per serving)

- Calories: 200 kcal
- Protein: 30g
- Fat: 3g
- Carbohydrates: 14g

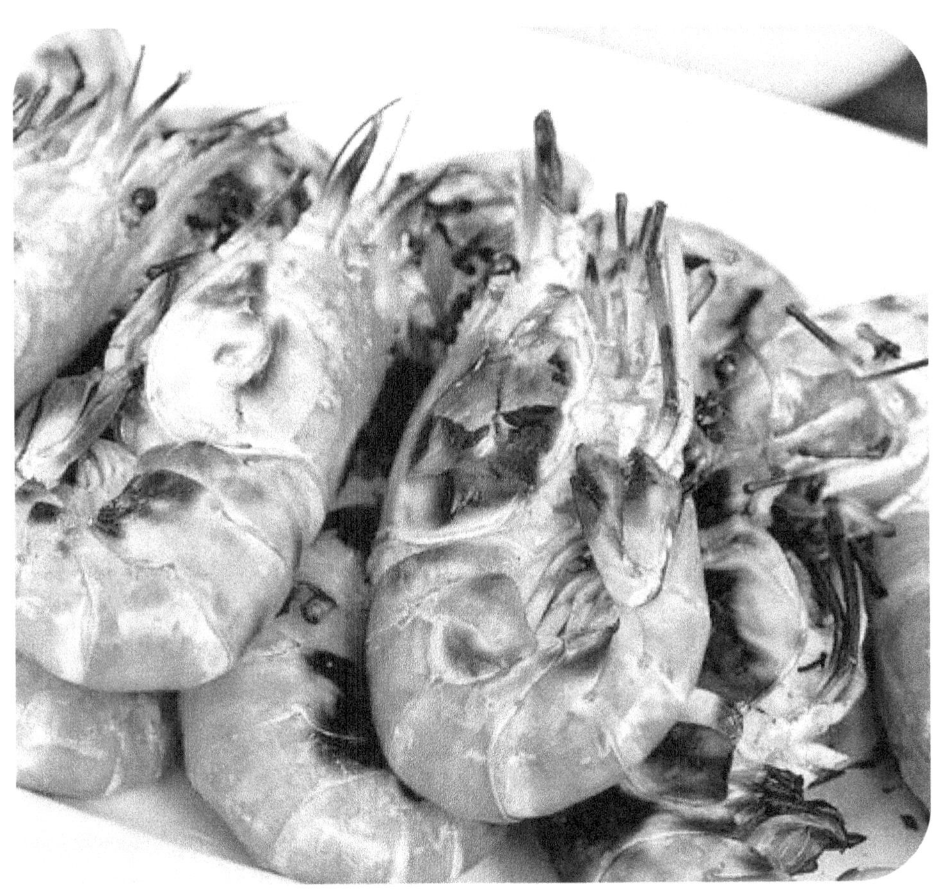

Tomato and Lentil Soup with Spinach

Preparation Time:

10 minutes

Cooking Time:

40 minutes

Number of Servings:

10

Ingredients

- 2 tablespoons extra virgin olive oil
- 3 carrots, diced
- 2-3 celery stalks, diced
- 1 large onion, diced
- 3-4 garlic cloves, minced
- 1 red bell pepper, diced
- 1 lb dried lentils
- 2 (about 1 pound) cans of diced Italian tomatoes with juice
- 4 cups vegetable or chicken broth
- 5 cups water
- 2 1/2 teaspoons Italian seasoning
- 4 pinches of kosher salt, divided
- Freshly ground black pepper, divided
- 10 oz fresh spinach
- Freshly grated Parmesan cheese, for serving

Instructions

1. First, start with the vegetables. In a big saucepan set over medium heat, warm the olive oil. Add minced garlic, red bell pepper, onion, and carrots, all chopped.

2. Toss with two pinches of salt and freshly ground black pepper. Vegetables should be tender and fragrant after 7 to 10 minutes of cooking.

3. Stir in the lentils, then mix them with the diced tomatoes, their juice, broth, and water. Give it two additional pinches of salt.

4. Cook the soup over medium-high heat, stirring occasionally, then turn it down to a simmer. Cook for 35 to 40 minutes, partially covered with a lid, stirring occasionally, until the soup thickens.

5. Taste the soup as it cooks, and, if needed, add additional water or salt and pepper. Though lentils will absorb a lot of liquid, the soup should be somewhat watery when done.

6. Stir in the spinach leaves until they wilt during the last five minutes of cooking.

7. Serve with freshly grated Parmesan cheese on top of the dishes. Cheers to your dinner!

Estimated Nutrition Information (per serving)

- Calories: 280 kcal
- Protein: 14g
- Fat: 3g
- Carbohydrates: 24g

Mini Meat Muffins with Vegetables

Preparation Time:

15 minutes

Cooking Time:

60 minutes

Number of Servings:

6

Ingredients

Meat Mixture:

- 600 grams ground meat (your choice!)
- 1/2 zucchini, diced
- 1 onion, chopped finely
- 1 red bell pepper, diced (optional: peas, string beans, carrots, or corn)
- 2 cloves garlic, minced
- 2 tablespoons vegetable oil
- 2 tablespoons breadcrumbs
- 100 grams grated hard cheese
- 2 eggs
- Salt and black pepper to taste
- Fresh herbs (optional)

Garnish:

- Fresh herbs (optional)
- Chopped vegetables (optional)

Instructions

1. Heat oil in a pan over medium heat. Saute the onion and garlic for 2 minutes until they begin to soften. Add the diced zucchini and bell pepper (and other vegetables if desired). Season with salt and herbs then cook for 5 minutes until they start to become tender. Allow cooling slightly.
2. Mix together the ground meat, cooled vegetables, eggs, breadcrumbs, salt, and black pepper in a large bowl.
3. Preheat oven to 400°F (200°C). Lightly grease a muffin tin.
4. Fill muffin cups with meat mixture, pressing down firmly (do not overfill). Bake for 40 minutes.
5. Sprinkle grated cheese on top of them about 10 minutes before it's done baking. Raise oven heat to high (or use a broiler) and place pan on the top rack to melt and brown cheese.
6. Now it's all done. serve hot as a main course or cold as an appetizer. Garnish with fresh herbs or chopped vegetables if you wish.

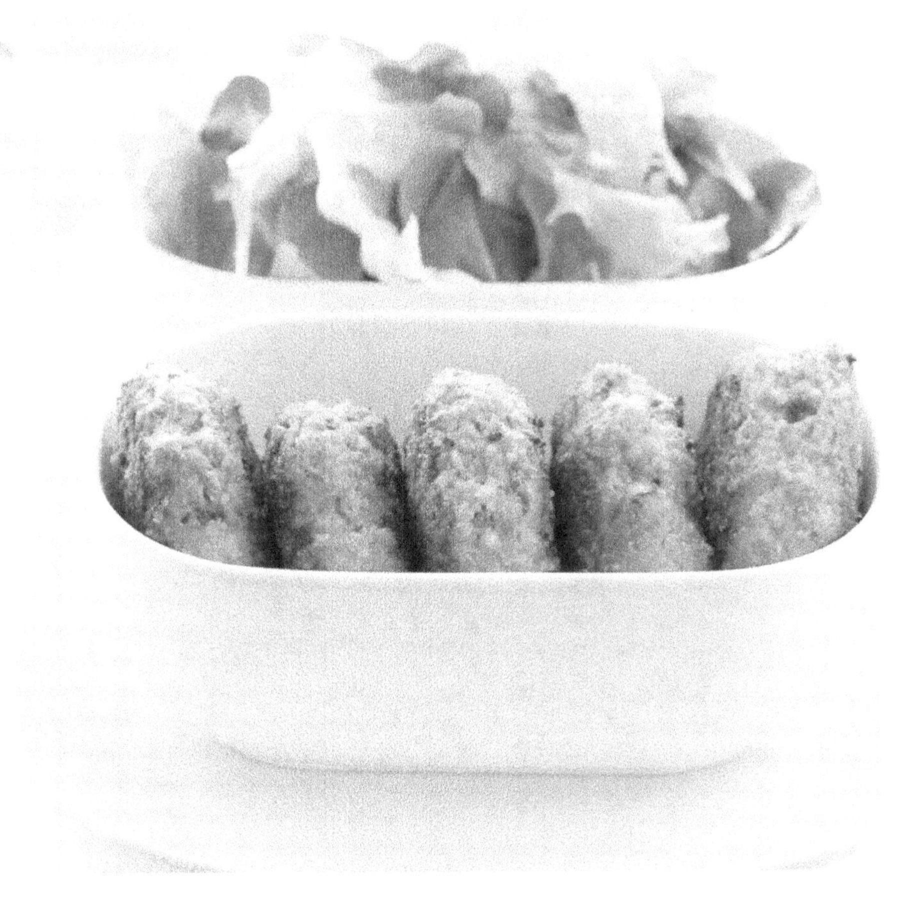

Spaghetti Squash Bolognese

Preparation Time:

20 minutes

Cooking Time:

50 minutes

Number of Servings:

4-5

Ingredients

For the Spaghetti Squash:

- 1 large spaghetti squash
- 1 Tbsp algae oil or avocado oil
- 1/4 tsp sea salt

Bolognese:

- 2 Tbsp algae oil or avocado oil
- 1/2 medium yellow onion, finely chopped
- 5 cloves garlic, minced
- 1 Tbsp dried oregano
- 1 Tbsp dried parsley
- 2 tsp paprika
- 2 tsp dried thyme
- 2 tsp dried rosemary
- 2 tsp dried basil
- 1/4 tsp cayenne pepper

- 1 lb grass-fed ground beef
- 1 tsp sea salt, to taste
- 1 (28-ounce) can crushed tomatoes
- 3 Tbsp tomato paste
- 2 tsp pure maple syrup (optional)

Instructions

Prepare the spaghetti squash

1. To roast, heat the oven to 415°F. Cut off both sides of this spaghetti squash, scoop out the seeds and pulp over a metal spoon.
2. Brush inside with olive oil from algae and sprinkle on sea salt. Place the cut side down on a baking sheet and cook for 45–50 minutes until very tender.
3. Take it off the stove and let it cool to a temperature you can handle. Using a fork, pull in strands that look like spaghetti and separate them into 2 to 4 bowls.

Make the Bolognese sauce

4. As you roast the squash, heat olive oil made from algae in a large skillet at medium heat.
5. Stir occasionally for about 8 minutes, until the onion is translucent. Add minced garlic and herbs (oregano through cayenne) and sauté for another 3 minutes.
6. Push the onions to one side of the skillet, then put in the ground beef. Let the beef brown undisturbed for about 3 minutes, flip over, and brown the other side for an additional 3 minutes.
7. Use a spatula to break the meat apart and stir everything together; at this point, do not fully cook the meat. Stir well after adding sea salt, crushed tomatoes, tomato paste, or real maple syrup, if desired.
8. Bring the sauce to a boil before reducing the heat to simmering mode, gently stirring for sometimes as long as half an hour or even sixty minutes.

9. Taste your sauce and add more salt if necessary!

Serve:

- Ladle the Bolognese sauce over the roasted spaghetti squash strands and garnish with fresh basil.

Estimated Nutrition Information (per serving)

- Calories: 384 kcal
- Protein: 29g
- Fat: 20g
- Carbohydrates: 23g

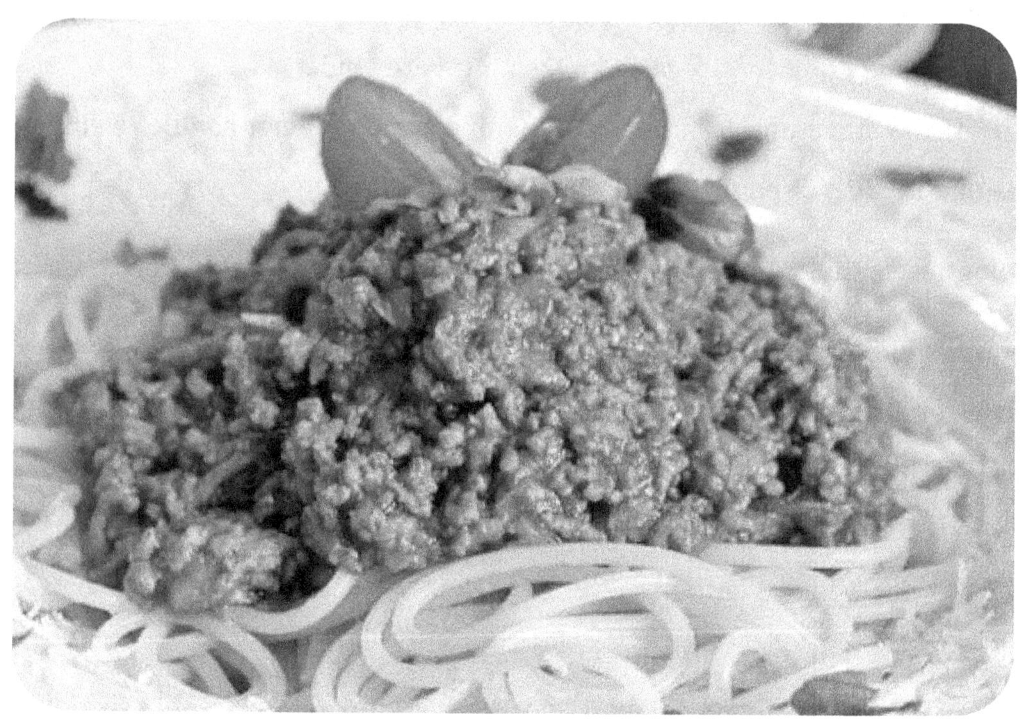

Spaghetti Squash with Chicken, Mushrooms, Garlic, And Kale

Preparation Time:

20 minutes

Cooking Time:

1 hour

Number of Servings:

3

Ingredients

- 1 medium-sized spaghetti squash, roasted
- 2 Tbsp avocado oil (or olive oil)
- 1 medium yellow onion, thinly sliced
- 5 large garlic cloves, minced
- 3 cups baby Portobello mushrooms, chopped into sixths
- 2 tsp fresh thyme, chopped
- 2 large chicken breasts, sliced into strips (about 1 to 1.5 lbs)
- 1/2 cup chicken broth
- 4 cups kale leaves
- Zest of 1 lemon
- 1/2 tsp sea salt, to taste

Instructions

Roast the spaghetti squash

1. Put your oven at 400°F (200°C). Then slice the spaghetti squash lengthwise and remove the seeds. Sprinkle some sea salt on it, then lightly coat it with avocado oil.
2. Take a baking sheet and place the halves facing down. Bake them for about 40–50 minutes, or until they become tender. Remove from the oven and cool.

Prepare the rest of the dish:

3. During the roasting process, heat two tablespoons of avocado oil in a skillet over medium-high heat. Add sliced onion to this mixture, stir, and fry occasionally for approximately fifteen to twenty minutes until deeply browned or almost caramelized.
4. You can turn down the heat to low if the slice starts burning and add some chicken stock to deglaze the pan.
5. Also, add minced garlic, chopped mushrooms, and sliced chicken to the pan. Allow these mushrooms to cook until soft, as well as the chicken, for up to 5 minutes, until browned.
6. The poultry broth is then poured into it while adding lemon zest, fresh thyme, and sea salt. Bring it gently to a boil, then put the kale leaves inside the skillet. Once covered, you have to let it cook for about 35 minutes until the chicken is fully cooked and the kale has wilted.

Combine everything

7. When spaghetti squash becomes cool enough so that you can handle it comfortably, scrape out its strands using a fork and place it in a large bowl.
8. Add the chicken and vegetable mixture to the bowl with the spaghetti squash and toss everything together until well combined. Taste and adjust the seasoning with more sea salt and/or lemon juice if needed.

Enjoy your meal.

Estimated Nutrition Information (per serving)

- Calories: 359 kcal
- Protein: 42g
- Fat: 15g
- Carbohydrates: 20g

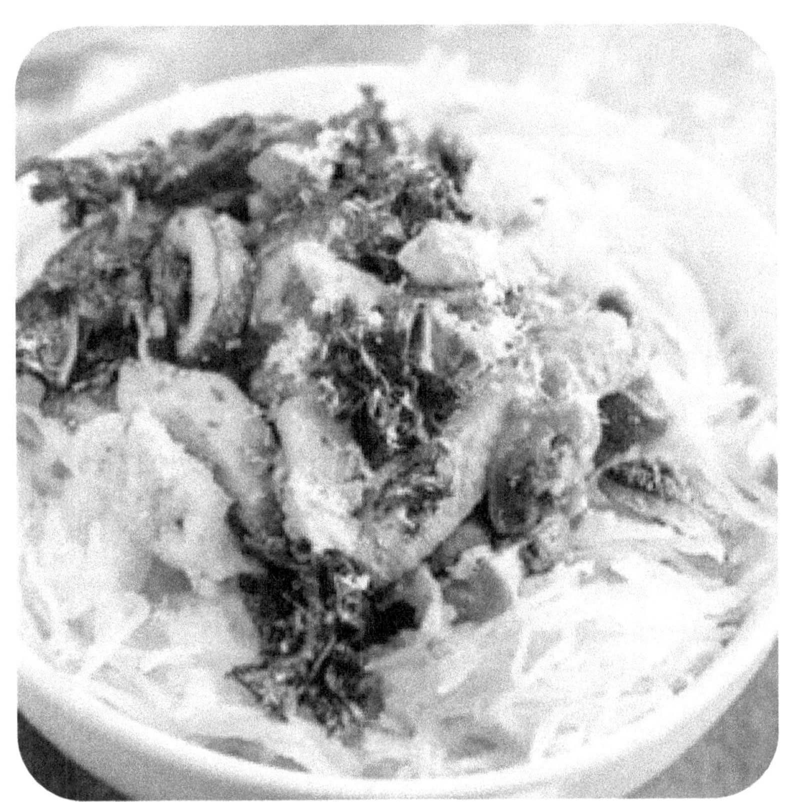

Chicken Pesto with Spaghetti Squash

Preparation Time:

20 minutes

Cooking Time:

1 hour

Number of Servings:

5

Ingredients

Spaghetti Squash:

- 1 large spaghetti squash
- 2 Tbsp avocado oil
- Pinch of sea salt

Chicken:

- 1 1/2 lbs boneless, skinless chicken thighs, chopped
- 1 Tbsp avocado oil
- 1 tsp paprika
- 1 tsp garlic powder
- Pinch of sea salt

Pesto:

- 2 cups fresh basil leaves
- 2/3 cup raw pumpkin seeds (pepitas)
- 2/3 cup avocado oil
- 1 large garlic clove
- 1 cup grated Parmesan cheese (optional)

Instructions

1. **Roast the Spaghetti Squash**: Preheat your oven to 400°F (200°C). Slice the spaghetti squash lengthwise and empty out its seeds. Sprinkle salt over the flesh and drizzle avocado oil on it. Then, arrange halves of the squash, cut side down, on a baking sheet. Put into an oven for about 40-50 minutes or until tender when pricked with a fork. Take it out of the oven and allow cooling.

2. **Make the Pesto (While Squash Roasts)**: In a food processor combine basil leaves, pumpkin seeds and garlic clove. Roughly chop by pulsating several times together. Keep adding Avocado oil slowly while motor is still running until pesto gets desired thickness that may be smooth or slightly chunky then add Parmesan cheese if using and blend well.

3. **Cook the Chicken**: Heat a large skillet over medium-high heat; add 1 tbs of avocado oil; season chopped chicken with salt, paprika, and garlic powder; put in pan without stirring for 3 minutes to brown; break up lumps by stirring once in three minutes for another three minutes; stir once more then cover pan while cooking additional 2-5 minutes until chicken is done.

4. **Assemble and Serve**: As soon as the squash is cool and comfortable to handle, use a fork to scrape out the spaghetti-like strands into large bowl then add prepared pesto tossing everything gently together so that each strand is coated evenly with it. Add the cooked chicken and any leftover pan drippings from the chicken to the bowl and toss to combine. Taste and, if necessary, add extra salt to adjust the seasoning.

Estimated Nutrition Information (per serving)

- Calories: 438 kcal
- Protein: 28g
- Fat: 22g
- Carbohydrates: 10g

Oven-Baked Salmon with Sautéed Mushrooms and Steamed Broccoli

Preparation Time:

10 minutes

Cooking Time:

20 minutes

Number of Servings:

4

Ingredients

Salmon:

- 4 salmon fillets (about 6 oz each)
- 2 Tbsp olive oil
- 1 lemon, sliced
- 1 tsp sea salt
- 1/2 tsp black pepper

Sautéed Mushrooms:

- 2 Tbsp olive oil
- 3 cups mushrooms, sliced
- 3 garlic cloves, minced
- 1 tsp fresh thyme, chopped (optional)
- 1/2 tsp sea salt
- 1/4 tsp black pepper

Steamed Broccoli:

- 4 cups broccoli florets

- 1/2 lemon, juiced

- 1/4 tsp sea salt

Instructions

1. **Preheat the Oven:** Your oven should be heated to 400° Fahrenheit (200°C).

2. **Get the Salmon Ready:** With parchment paper, line your baking sheet. Place the salmon fillets on the prepared sheet. Drizzle olive oil over them and sprinkle with sea salt and black pepper before putting some lemon slices on top of each fillet.

3. **Bake the Salmon:** Put in the oven and bake for 12-15 minutes or until when you tell that it is cooked by pricking it with a fork easily.

4. **Sauté the Mushrooms (While Salmon Bakes):** In a large skillet, heat olive oil over medium heat, add sliced mushrooms, and cook until they begin to brown about 5-7 minutes.

5. **Add Flavor to the Mushrooms:** Stir in minced garlic, fresh thyme if using, sea salt, and black pepper. Cook for another 2-3 minutes so that mushrooms become tender and fragrant.

6. **Steam the Broccoli (While Mushrooms Sauté):** Fill a pot with water, and put it on heat until boiling point. Afterward, place a steamer basket above it then place broccoli florets in there before covering again so that it can steam for roughly five to seven minutes till when its color turns green but not pale.

7. **Finishing Touches:** Take out Broccoli from the cooking pot, drizzle lemon juice over it, then sprinkle some sea salt too.

8. **Serve:** Arrange baked salmon fillets alongside sautéed mushrooms and steamed broccoli on plates. Enjoy your tasty healthy meal!

Estimated Nutrition Information (per serving)

- Calories: 379 kcal

- Protein: 34g

- Fat: 14g

- Carbohydrates: 11g

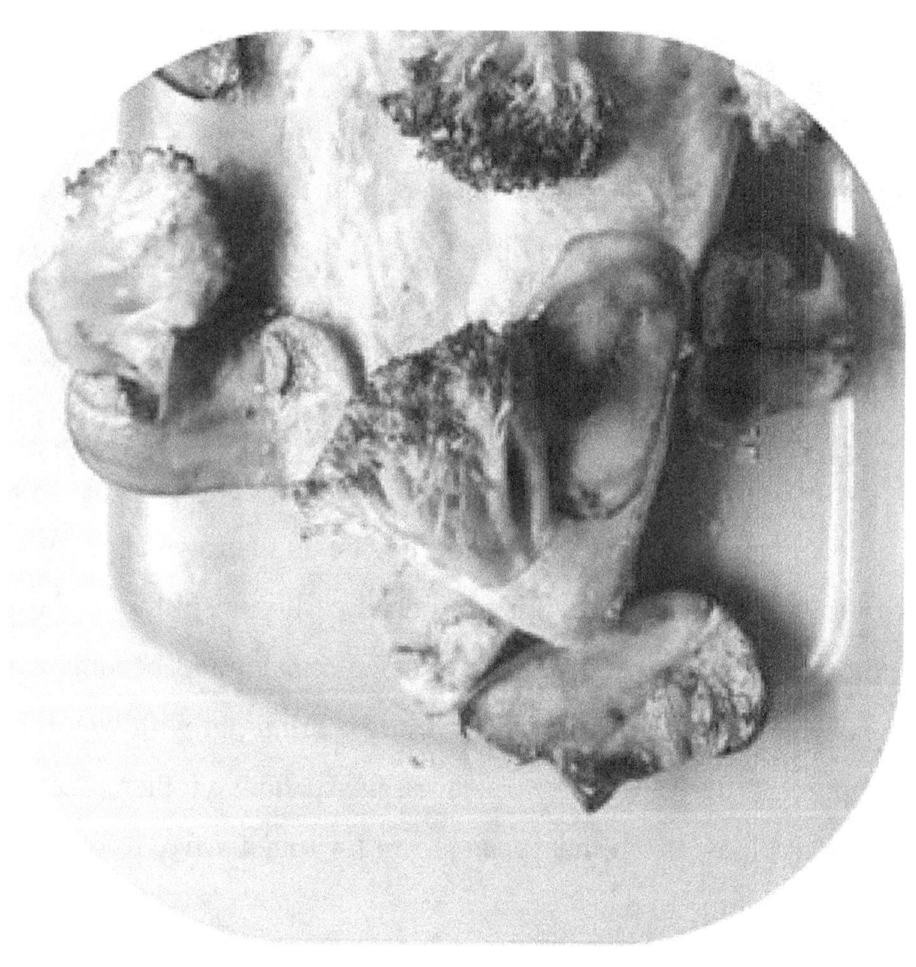

Oven-Baked Salmon with Sweet Potato & Steamed Green Beans

Preparation Time:

10 minutes

Cooking Time:

25 minutes

Number of Servings:

4

Ingredients

Vegetables:

- 1 pound of potatoes, cut into quarters
- 2 tablespoons olive oil
- ¾ teaspoon sea salt (divided in half)
- ¼ teaspoon black pepper (divided in half)

Salmon:

- 4 (6-ounce) salmon fillets

Flavorful Extras:

- 4 tablespoons melted ghee or avocado oil
- 4 cloves garlic, minced
- 2 tablespoons chopped fresh parsley
- 2 tablespoons fresh lemon juice
- 1 pound trimmed green beans

For garnish:

- Lemon slices (optional)

Instructions

---

1. **Preheat Oven:** Preheat your oven to 400°F (200°C).

2. **Prepare the Potatoes:** Toss the quartered potatoes with 1/4 teaspoon black pepper, 1/2 teaspoon sea salt, and olive oil in a bowl. Arrange them on a big baking sheet so that they are in a uniform layer. Roast for 13 to 15 minutes, or until they begin to color slightly and are just tender.

3. **Prepare Salmon:** Put the potatoes to one side and take the baking sheet out of the oven. In the middle of the sheet, arrange the salmon fillets.

4. **Make the Butter Mixture:** In a small bowl, melt the ghee or avocado oil. Whisk in the minced garlic, chopped parsley, and lemon juice. Reserve 1-1/2 tablespoons of this mixture and set it aside.

5. **Season the Salmon:** Rub the salmon fillets evenly with the remaining butter mixture.

6. **Add Green Beans:** On the other side of the baking sheet, add the green beans. Toss them with the reserved 1-1/2 tablespoons of the butter mixture. Season everything with the remaining sea salt and black pepper.

7. **Bake:** Place the baking sheet back in the oven and bake for a further 10 minutes or so, or until the salmon is cooked through and the potatoes are golden and soft. Check the salmon's doneness using an instant-read thermometer; it's done when it hits 145°F (63°C). For the final two to three minutes of cooking, you can broil the pan to get further browning.

8. **Serve:** With lemon slices as a garnish, serve the baked salmon with the potatoes and green beans.

Estimated Nutrition Information (per serving)

- Calories: 438 kcal
- Protein: 38g
- Fat: 22g
- Carbohydrates: 20g

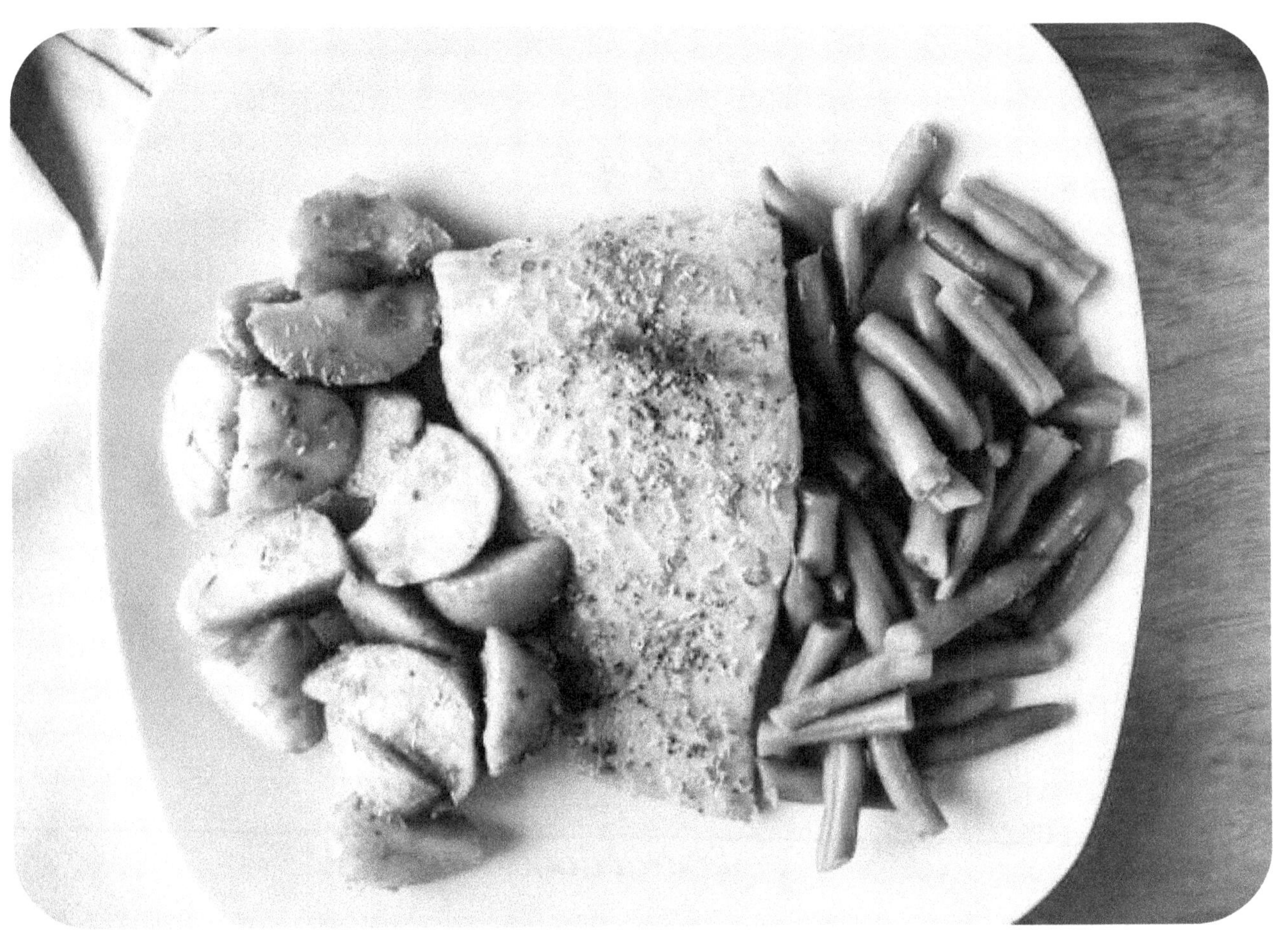

Creamy Shrimp and Broccoli Pasta

Preparation Time:

10 minutes

Cooking Time:

20 minutes

Number of Servings:

4

Ingredients

- 8 ounces of whole wheat pasta shells (boiled and drained)
- 3 tablespoons avocado oil, or ghee
- 2 tsp minced garlic
- 2 tablespoons almond flour
- 3 cups unsweetened almond milk
- 2/3 cup nutritional yeast or grated Parmesan cheese
- 1–2 tsp sea salt, to taste
- 1/4 teaspoon ground or 1/2 teaspoon cracked black pepper
- 1 pound of medium or big shrimp. (Peel and deveined)
- 2 tsp olive oil
- 3 cups broccoli florets and one cup water

Instructions

1. In a large frying pan set over medium heat, warm the olive oil. Stirring now and again for 4 to 6 minutes, until they solidify and turn pinkish white. To keep it warm, spoon it onto a platter and cover.

2. In the same skillet, you would then add the broccoli florets and water. Cook with the pan covered for 4 to 6 minutes, or until the potatoes are crispy but still soft. After draining any extra liquid, put the broccoli and shrimp aside.

3. To make the creamy sauce, return the pan to medium heat and add the ghee or avocado oil. When melted, add minced garlic and heat through, stirring, for around a minute. Then pour the melted fat over the almond flour, whisking constantly until everything is mixed. Pour in some almond milk gradually until the mixture is creamy and smooth.

4. Keep heating and whisking until everything is properly blended and the cheese melts fully. you can taste the sauce to see whether the seasoning is ok or not.

5. Toss in the cooked and drained pasta shells, steamed broccoli, and cooked shrimp into the creamy sauce and mix them thoroughly.

6. Top with additional nutritional yeast or Parmesan cheese and serve immediately.

Estimated Nutrition Information (per serving)

- Calories: 451 kcal
- Protein: 26g
- Fat: 19g
- Carbohydrates: 45g

Shrimp and Veggie Cauliflower Fried Rice

Preparation Time:

25 minutes

Cooking Time:

25 minutes

Number of Servings:

4

Ingredients

- 2 big eggs
- 1/4 cup sesame oil.
- 3 cups broiled cauliflower
- 1 pound Large shrimp, peeled and deveined
- 3 cups chopped broccoli florets
- 1 thinly cut medium red bell pepper (approximately one cup)
- 3 chopped garlic cloves
- 3 teaspoons tamari or reduced-sodium soy sauce
- 2 tablespoons water
- 1 tsp rice vinegar
- 1/2 teaspoon of black pepper.

Instructions

1. In a big, flat-bottomed wok or heavy pan set over high heat, warm two tablespoons of sesame oil. Add the beaten eggs and cook, stirring, for about 30 seconds, until one side sets. Cook, flipping, for an additional fifteen seconds, or until done. Transfer the eggs onto a chopping board and chop them into 1/2-inch pieces.

2. Add two tablespoons of sesame oil to the pan and heat it on high. Evenly distribute the riced cauliflower across the pan and cook, uncovered, for three to four minutes, until just faintly browned. Transfer to a plate.

3. Add two more tablespoons of sesame oil to the pan and heat it on high. Cook the shrimp for around 3 minutes, stirring often, until they are just opaque. Spoon onto the platter beside the cauliflower.

4. Add the remaining two teaspoons of sesame oil to the pan and heat it over high. Shred the garlic, then add broccoli and red bell pepper. Cook for 4 to 5 minutes, stirring occasionally, until the vegetables are just barely browned.

5. Add the water, rice vinegar, soy sauce (or tamari), and ground black pepper. Boil the mixture for 30 seconds. Take off the heat and thoroughly mix in the shrimp, cauliflower, and reserved eggs. Serve immediately.

Estimated Nutrition Information (per serving)

- Calories: 309 kcal
- Protein: 31g
- Fat: 15g
- Carbohydrates: 10g

Shrimp Scampi with Whole-Wheat Pasta

Preparation Time:

25 minutes

Cooking Time:

20 minutes

Number of Servings:

4

Ingredients

- 8 ounces cappellini or whole wheat spaghetti
- 3 tablespoons olive oil,
- 1 medium thinly sliced red bell pepper
- 5 big garlic cloves (chopped)
- 1/2 cup low-sodium chicken broth or white wine
- 1/8 tsp, or to taste, red pepper flakes
- 1 1/2 pounds, Large shrimp, peeled and deveined
- 2 tablespoons freshly squeezed lemon juice
- 1/3 cup fresh parsley, chopped
- Salt and freshly ground black pepper

Instructions

1. Heat up a big saucepan of salted water. Put the whole-wheat pasta in it and boil it according to the pack's instructions. Drain and keep aside.

2. As you cook the pasta, heat 3 tablespoons of extra-virgin olive oil in a large non-stick frying pan over medium-high heat. Add thinly sliced red bell pepper and sauté for about 2 minutes, stirring once in a while. Add minced garlic and continue to stir for another minute.
3. Pour white wine (or low-sodium chicken broth) into the skillet along with red pepper flakes. Simmer this mixture until it reduces slightly, which takes around one minute.
4. Put the shrimp that have been peeled and deveined into the skillet. Stir constantly till they turn pink and are opaque at their centers, approximately three minutes.
5. Next, remove the skillet from the heat and add freshly squeezed lemon juice to it.
6. Now combine drained pasta, shrimp mixture, and chopped parsley in a large serving bowl. Add salt and freshly ground black pepper to taste then toss everything together well so that it is evenly mixed.
7. Serve immediately garnished with more parsley if desired.

Estimated Nutrition Information (per serving)

- Calories: 480 kcal
- Protein: 44g
- Fat: 12g
- Carbohydrates: 40g

Chapter 8 - Snacks Recipes

Sliced Apples with Peanut Butter

Preparation Time:

5 minutes

Cooking Time:

0 minutes

Number of Servings:

1

Ingredients

- 1 medium apple, any kind
- 2 tsp creamy or chunky peanut butter

Instructions

1. First, the apple should be well-washed.
2. Cut it into little cubes, and circular slices
3. Serve the apple slices in a little dish or platter.
4. Set down two teaspoons of peanut butter next to the apple for dipping.

Notes

- This delicious snack is considered both vegan and gluten-free.
- Any leftover apple slices and peanut butter should be kept in an airtight container and refrigerated for 2-3 days.

Estimated Nutrition Information (per serving)

- Calories: 286 kcal
- Protein: 9g
- Fat: 15g
- Carbohydrates: 30g
- Sodium: 139mg
- Potassium: 375mg
- Fiber: 6g
- Sugar: 19g
- Vitamin A: 98 IU
- Vitamin C: 8 mg
- Calcium: 27 mg
- Iron: 1 mg

No-Bake Protein Bars

Preparation Time:

15 minutes

Cooking Time:

0 minutes

Number of Servings:

12

Ingredients

- 1 1/2 cups rolled oats
- 1 cup protein powder (preferably low in sugar)
- 1/2 cup almond butter or peanut butter (no added sugar)
- 1/4 cup honey or maple syrup
- 1/4 cup unsweetened almond milk
- 1/4 cup chia seeds
- 1/4 cup chopped nuts (almonds, walnuts, or any other preferred choice)
- 1/4 cup unsweetened shredded coconut
- 1 tsp vanilla extract
- 1/2 tsp ground cinnamon
- A pinch of sea salt

Instructions

1. In a large mixing bowl, combine what I like to call the dry ingredients; rolled oats, protein powder, chia seeds, chopped almonds, shredded coconut, crushed cinnamon, and sea salt, and thoroughly mix them.

2. Now mix the almond butter and honey (or maple syrup) and gently reheat them in a separate microwave-safe dish for 20 to 30 seconds.

3. Add the almond milk and vanilla essence, mixing thoroughly.

4. Pour the wet ingredients into the dry ones and stir until a thick dough forms and everything is uniformly combined.

5. Set parchment paper into an 8 by 8-inch baking dish. Spoon the mixture into the dish, then use a spatula or your hands to push it down firmly and evenly to form a level, even layer.

6. Give the dish two hours or more in the refrigerator to firm up the bars.

7. Cut the bars into 12 equal-sized pieces after removing them from the dish when they are hard.

Notes

- When stored in an airtight container, the bars can last up to a week in the refrigerator.

Estimated Nutrition Information (per serving)

- Calories: 199 kcal
- Protein: 11g
- Fat: 8g
- Carbohydrates: 18g
- Fiber: 4g

Sliced Apples with Almond Butter

Preparation Time:

5 minutes

Cooking Time:

0 minutes

Number of Servings:

1

Ingredients

- 1 medium or large apple
- 1 or 2 tsp smooth almond butter

Instructions

1. First, the apple should be well-washed.
2. Cut it into little cubes, and circular slices
3. Serve the apple slices in a little dish or platter.
4. Set down two teaspoons of almond butter next to the apple for dipping.

Estimated Nutrition Information (per serving)

- Calories: 186 kcal
- Protein: 8g
- Fat: 8g
- Carbohydrates: 25g
- Vitamin A: 98 IU
- Vitamin C: 8 mg
- Calcium: 27 mg

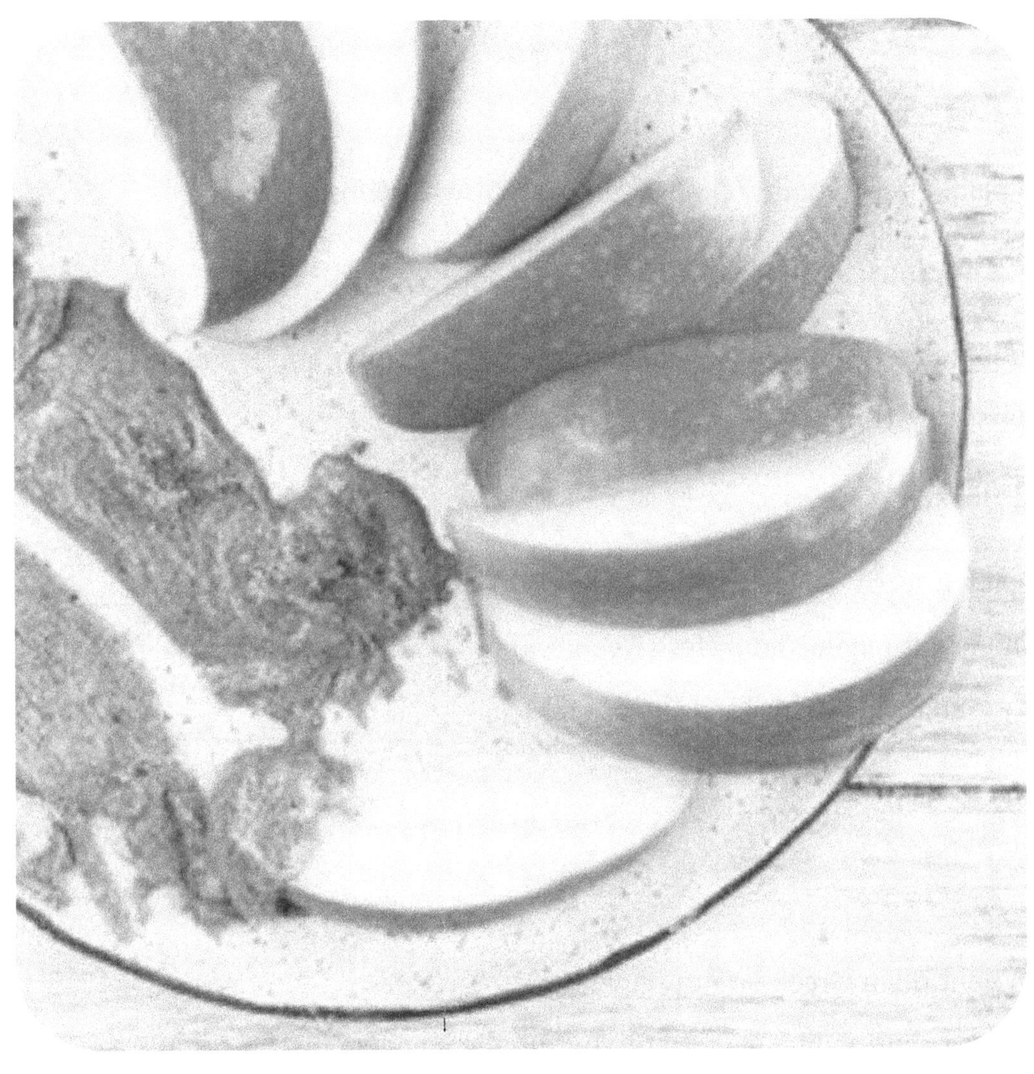

Greek Yogurt with Nuts

Preparation Time:

5 minutes

Cooking Time:

0 minutes

Number of Servings:

1

Ingredients

- 1 cup plain Greek yogurt (choose full-fat or low-fat, unsweetened)

Crunchy Toppings:

- ¼ cup mixed nuts (almonds, walnuts, cashews, or your choice), roughly chopped
- Fresh berries (your choice)

Optional Boosters:

- 1 Tbsp chia seeds or flaxseeds (for extra fiber)
- 1 tsp honey or maple syrup (for sweetness)
- ¼ tsp ground cinnamon (for a flavor kick)

Instructions

1. Spoon your plain Greek yogurt into a bowl.
2. Cover the yogurt with a handful of your preferred chopped mixed nuts.
3. You may add a sprinkling of flaxseeds or chia seeds for extra fiber.

4. For extra sweetness, drizzle with a little amount of honey or maple syrup, and then top with ground cinnamon.
5. You may also top with your preferred berries.
6. Grab a spoon and enjoy this tasty and healthy snack.

Estimated Nutrition Information (per serving)

- Calories: 290 kcal

- Protein: 20g

- Fat: 14g

- Carbohydrates: 15g

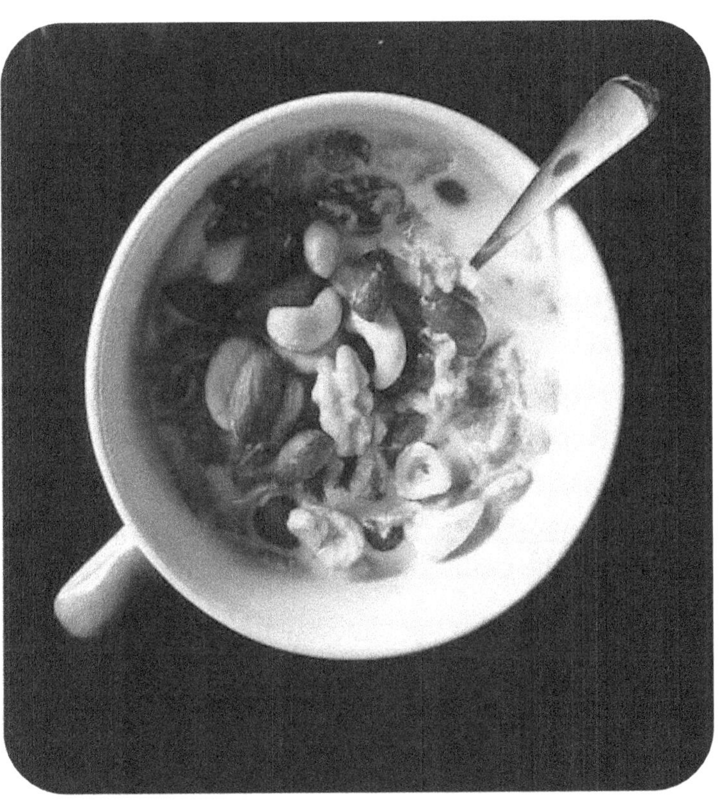

Whipped Cottage Cheese

Preparation Time:

10 minutes

Cooking Time:

0 minutes

Number of Servings:

2

Ingredients

- 1 cup full- or low-fat cottage cheese
- One teaspoon vanilla extract
- 1-2 tablespoons of unsweetened cocoa powder (optional for adding chocolate flavor)
- 1-2 tablespoons of sweetener (stevia, erythritol, or monk fruit; taste and adjust)
- Dark chocolate shavings or fresh berries as a garnish (optional).

Instructions

1. Put the cottage cheese in a blender or food processor.
2. Mix the cottage cheese with the sugar, vanilla extract, and chocolate powder (if you choose to use it).

3. Blend everything together until it is creamy and smooth and use a spatula to scrape down the sides as required.

4. Spoon the cottage cheese into serving dishes.

5. If preferred, sprinkle some dark chocolate shavings or fresh berries on top.

6. Serve right away and savor this high-protein, low-carb snack.

Estimated Nutrition Information (per serving)

- Calories: 150kcal

- Carbohydrates: 5g

- Protein: 13g

- Fat: 5g

Cucumber Hummus

Preparation Time:

10 minutes

Cooking Time:

0 minutes

Number of Servings:

2

Ingredients

- 1 cup English seedless cucumber, chopped
- 1 garlic clove, chopped
- 15-ounce can of chickpeas, drained and rinsed
- 1 tablespoon lemon juice
- 1 tablespoon olive oil
- 1/2 teaspoon salt
- 1/4 cup plus 2 tablespoons tahini
- 1/4 teaspoon cayenne pepper
- 1 tablespoon fresh dill, chopped
- 1 tablespoon fresh parsley, chopped

Instructions

1. For the hummus, add your chickpeas, diced cucumber, garlic, tahini, lemon juice, olive oil, salt, and cayenne pepper to a food processor and process till everything is smooth.

2. Next, add chopped parsley and dill to the hummus and stir. Add the herbs and pulse a few times to allow the flavors to combine.

3. Now, transfer the hummus to a serving bowl and place it in the fridge to chill for at least an hour.

4. Spread the hummus over your preferred vegetables or pita bread, and eat it cold or at room temperature.

Estimated Nutrition Information (per serving)

- Calories: 120 kcal
- Carbohydrates: 8g
- Protein: 6g
- Fat: 5g
- Fiber: 4g

Tuna Salad with Greek Yogurt

Preparation Time:

5 minutes

Cooking Time:

0 minutes

Number of Servings:

4

Ingredients

- 24 ounces of canned tuna (two 12-ounce cans packed in water)
- 1 clove garlic, minced
- Juice of 1/2 small lemon
- 1 teaspoon red pepper flakes (optional)
- 1 tablespoon Dijon mustard
- 1 dill pickle, finely diced
- 1 stalk celery, finely chopped
- 1 small red onion, minced
- 1/2 teaspoon salt
- 1/2 teaspoon black pepper
- 1/2 cup Greek yogurt
- 1/4 cup mayonnaise

Instructions

1. The canned tuna should first be completely drained before being flaked into tiny pieces using a fork.

2. Minced garlic, lemon juice, salt, black pepper, Greek yogurt, mayonnaise, red pepper flakes (if used), and Dijon mustard should all be well mixed together in a big mixing basin.

3. Now add the diced dill pickle, chopped celery, minced red onion, and flaked tuna to the bowl. Stir all the ingredients thoroughly until they are well combined.

4. Serve the tuna salad right away, or refrigerate it for up to 3–4 days in an airtight container.

Estimated Nutrition Information (per serving)

- Calories: 250 kcal
- Carbohydrates: 8g
- Protein: 36g
- Fat: 10g
- Fiber: 4g

Tuna Salad with Crackers

Preparation Time:

10 minutes

Cooking Time:

0 minutes

Number of Servings:

6

Ingredients

- 5 tablespoons mayonnaise
- 1 tsp minced onion
- 1 can (6 oz) tuna
- A dash of ground black pepper
- A dash of salt
- 1 pack of snack crackers
- 2 tsp minced celery
- 1 tsp superfine mustard powder

Instructions

1. Mix the drained tuna, minced onion, and minced celery in a bowl.

2. Furthermore, mayonnaise and mustard powder are to be added to the mixture of tuna. Stir all these ingredients thoroughly until they perfectly blend. Salt and ground black pepper can then be sprinkled to taste.

3. Now, cover the dish with a lid and keep it in the refrigerator for at least one hour to allow flavors to blend properly.

4. When serving, each cracker receives one tablespoon of tuna salad; then stack them on a plate for eating right away.

Estimated Nutrition Information (per serving)

- Calories: 140 kcal
- Carbohydrates: 6g
- Protein: 10g
- Fat: 8g
- Saturated Fat: 1.5g
- Sodium: 228mg

Chapter 9 - Smoothie Recipes

Refreshing Liver Detox Smoothie

This vibrant smoothie is packed with ingredients that detoxify and support liver health

Preparation Time:

10 minutes

Cooking Time:

Number of Servings:

1

Ingredients

- 1 ripe banana (or ½ cup chopped papaya for a tropical twist)
- ½ green apple, cored and chopped
- 1 medium carrot, peeled and chopped
- Handful of baby spinach
- ¼-inch piece of turmeric root, peeled
- 1 tablespoon chopped fresh parsley
- 3 walnut halves
- 2 tablespoons hemp protein powder
- ½ lemon, juiced
- Pinch of cinnamon (optional)
- ¾ cup unsweetened almond milk (or orange juice for a sweeter option)

Instructions

- Simply add all ingredients to a blender.

- Blend until smooth and creamy.

- Taste and adjust sweetness with additional cinnamon or a touch of honey if desired.

Estimated Nutrition Information (per serving)

- Calories: 217

- Carbohydrates: 41g

- Protein: 6g

- Fat: 3g

- Fiber: 9g

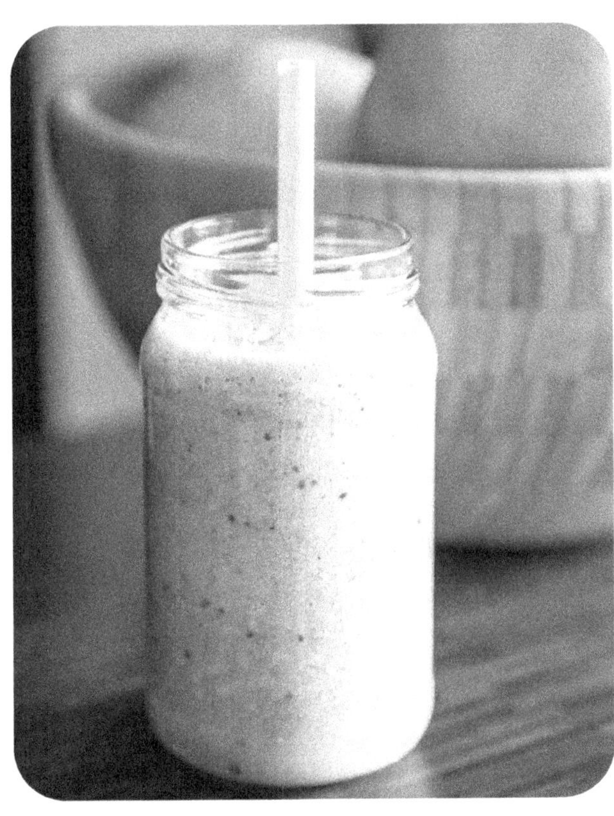

5-Minute Peanut Butter and Banana Smoothie

Preparation Time:

5 minutes

Cooking Time:

0 minutes

Number of Servings:

1

Ingredients

Base:

- 1 cup frozen ripe banana slices (about 1 medium banana)
- ⅓ cup rolled oats (use certified gluten-free oats if needed)
- ¾ to 1 cup unsweetened almond milk (or your preferred plant-based milk)
- 2-3 tablespoons peanut butter

Optional Add-Ins:

- Handful of baby spinach leaves
- 1 tablespoon flaxseed meal or hemp seeds (for extra nutrients)
- 1-2 teaspoons honey, maple syrup, or a pitted Medjool date (for sweetness)
- ¼ teaspoon ground cinnamon

Instructions

1. To start, put everything into a blender and process until creamy and smooth. To make the smoothie thinner, add extra almond milk. You can add additional bananas or oats for a thicker smoothie. If you want your peanut butter flavor to be stronger, then add more!

2. Enjoy your smoothie right away for the best texture and flavor. Better yet, freeze leftover smoothies in ice cube trays.

3. For a simple and delicious treat, blend frozen cubes with more plant-based milk later.

Estimated Nutrition Information (per serving)

- Calories: 426 kcal
- Carbohydrates: 54.6g
- Protein: 12.7g
- Fat: 20.4g

Carrot Cake Smoothie

Preparation Time:

5 minutes

Cooking Time:

0 minutes

Number of Servings:

1

Ingredients

- 1 large frozen banana
- 1 small chopped carrot
- 1/2 tsp vanilla extract
- 1 tsp fresh minced ginger
- Pinch of ground nutmeg
- 1/2 cup dairy-free milk (you can go for either one of these cashew, coconut, or almond)
- 1 scoop protein powder (optional)
- 1 pitted date (optional)
- 1/4 tsp ground cinnamon

Instructions

1. All ingredients—aside from protein powder, if using—should be blended until smooth. Keep adding milk to you reach your desired consistency

2. For additional flavor, add more date, ginger, or cinnamon. You can add protein powder if you want.

3. Serve immediately or, for an extra touch, top with hemp seeds, coconut, walnuts, or shredded carrot.

Estimated Nutrition Information (per serving)

- Calories: 170 kcal
- Carbohydrates: 30g
- Protein: 5 g
- Fat: 2 g

Note

For a perfect endomorph diet recipe, include protein powder for added satiety and limit the date (or omit it entirely) to control sugar content.

Energizing Green Smoothie Bowl

Preparation Time:

5 minutes

Cooking Time:

0 minutes

Number of Servings:

1

Ingredients

- 2 small frozen bananas
- ½ cup frozen blueberries
- 1 cup cauliflower (raw or steamed and frozen)
- ¾ - 1 cup unsweetened dairy-free milk (almond, coconut, etc.)
- 1 tsp maca powder (optional)
- 1 cup spinach
- 1 tsp ashwagandha powder (optional)
- 1 tsp spirulina powder (or use barley grass powder)
- 2 Tbsp hemp seeds
- 3 Tbsp peanut butter (or peanut butter powder for less fat)
- Grain-free granola (or omit for a grain-free option)
- Additional frozen blueberries

Instructions

1. All of the smoothie ingredients except toppings are blended in the high-speed blender at low/medium speed. If necessary, a blender wand may be used to mix everything together.
2. Add more dairy-free milk little by little until you find your right thickness- thicker for bowl and thinner for drink.
3. Taste it and add more peanut butter for density, banana for sweetness or spirulina/spinach to make it greener.
4. Put the smoothie into a bowl and garnish with preferred toppings if desired.

Estimated Nutrition Information (per serving)

- Calories: 385 kcal
- Carbohydrates: 40.8 g
- Protein: 15.6 g
- Fat: 19.7 g

Notes

- For protein and good fats, use peanut butter (or powder).
- Choose a grain-free substitute for the granola.

Protein Smoothie with Blueberries and Peanut Butter

Preparation Time:

5 minutes

Cooking Time:

0 minutes

Number of Servings:

1

Ingredients

1/2 cup frozen wild blueberries

1 large handful of organic spinach

1 scoop peanut butter protein powder

1 ripe banana, (already sliced and frozen)

½ - 1 cup dairy-free milk of choice (almond or cashew preferred)

1 Tbsp hemp or flax seeds (optional)

Instructions

1. Toss all your ingredients - frozen banana, blueberries, spinach, protein powder, and a half-cup of dairy-free milk - into a high-powered blender. If you choose to use hemp or flax seeds, add those in too. Blend everything on high until it's nice and creamy, scraping down the sides as needed for a smooth consistency.

2. Take a sip and see if your smoothie needs any tweaks. Craving more sweetness? Add some extra bananas. Want a stronger peanut butter flavor? Include more protein powder. Too thick? Blend in a little more dairy-free milk.

3. Pour your delicious creation into a glass and enjoy it right away. Leftovers? Stash them in the fridge (covered) for up to a day, but fresh is always best. You can also freeze leftover smoothies in ice cube trays for an easy future smoothie booster!

Estimated Nutrition Information (per serving)

- Calories: 388 kcal
- Carbohydrates: 47.6g
- Protein: 24.4g
- Fat: 14g

Oatmeal and Berries Smoothie

Preparation Time:

5 minutes

Cooking Time:

0 minutes

Number of Servings:

2

Ingredients

- 1/2 cup rolled oats
- 1/2 cup coconut water
- 1/2 cup blackberries
- 1/2 cup blueberries
- 1/2 cup strawberries
- 1/2 cup freshly squeezed orange juice
- 1/2 tsp coconut shavings (Toppings)

Instructions

1. Combine all the ingredients in a blender and blend until it's completely smooth.
2. Pour into glasses, top with coconut shavings, and enjoy while cold!

Estimated Nutrition Information (per serving)

- Calories: 164 kcal

- Carbohydrates: 34g

- Protein: 5g

- Fat: 2g

- Fiber: 6g

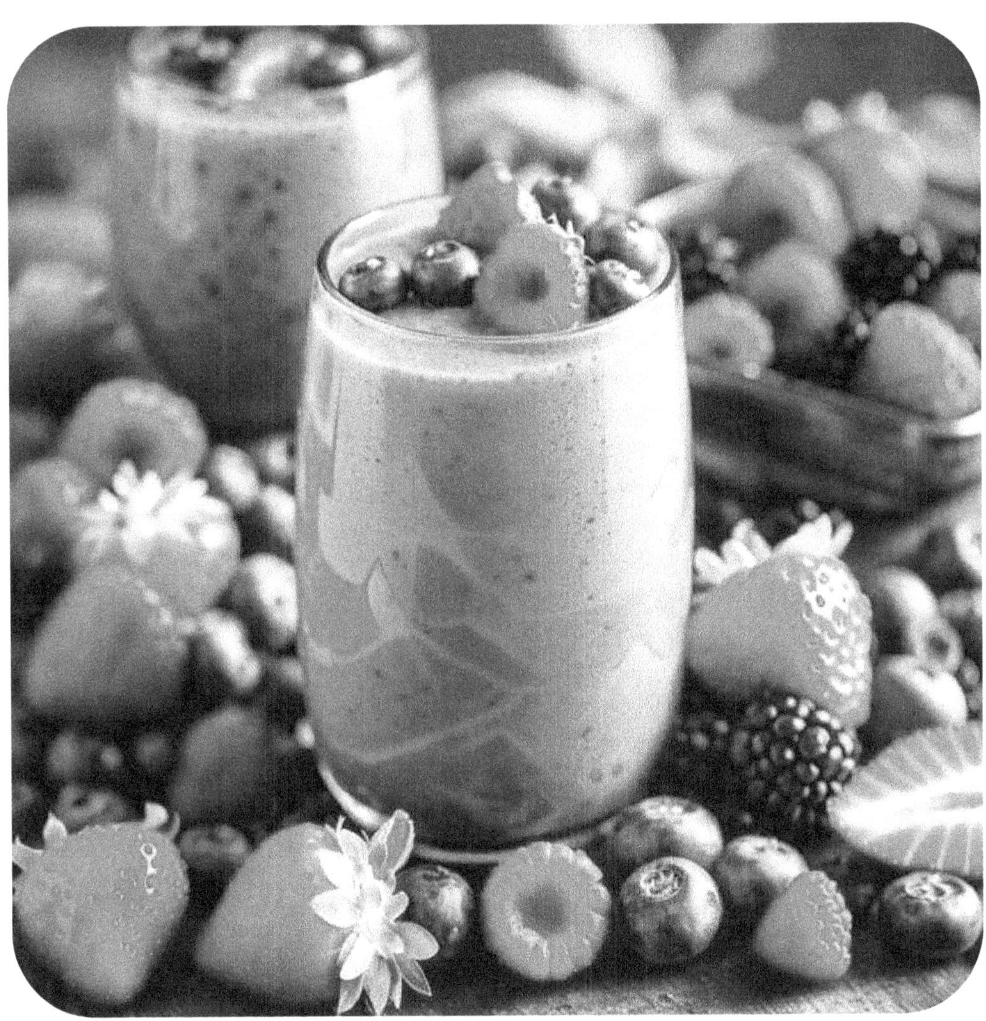

Almond and Zucchini Smoothie

Preparation Time:

5 minutes

Cooking Time:

0 minutes

Number of Servings:

2

Ingredients

- 1 small zucchini, chopped
- ¼ cup raw almonds
- 1 cup unsweetened almond milk
- 1 ripe banana, sliced and frozen
- 1 tablespoon almond butter
- 1 tablespoon chia seeds
- ½ teaspoon vanilla extract
- ¼ teaspoon ground cinnamon
- Ice cubes (optional, for a thicker consistency)

Instructions

1. Chop the zucchini and the banana if you forgot to slice it.
2. Combine all ingredients in a blender and blend on high until smooth and creamy.
3. Although this is optional, you can adjust the consistency by adding ice cubes for a thicker smoothie and blending again.
4. Pour the smoothie into a glass and enjoy it immediately.

Estimated Nutrition Information (per serving)

- Calories: 320 kcal
- Carbohydrates: 32g
- Protein: 8g
- Fat: 18g
- Fiber: 9g

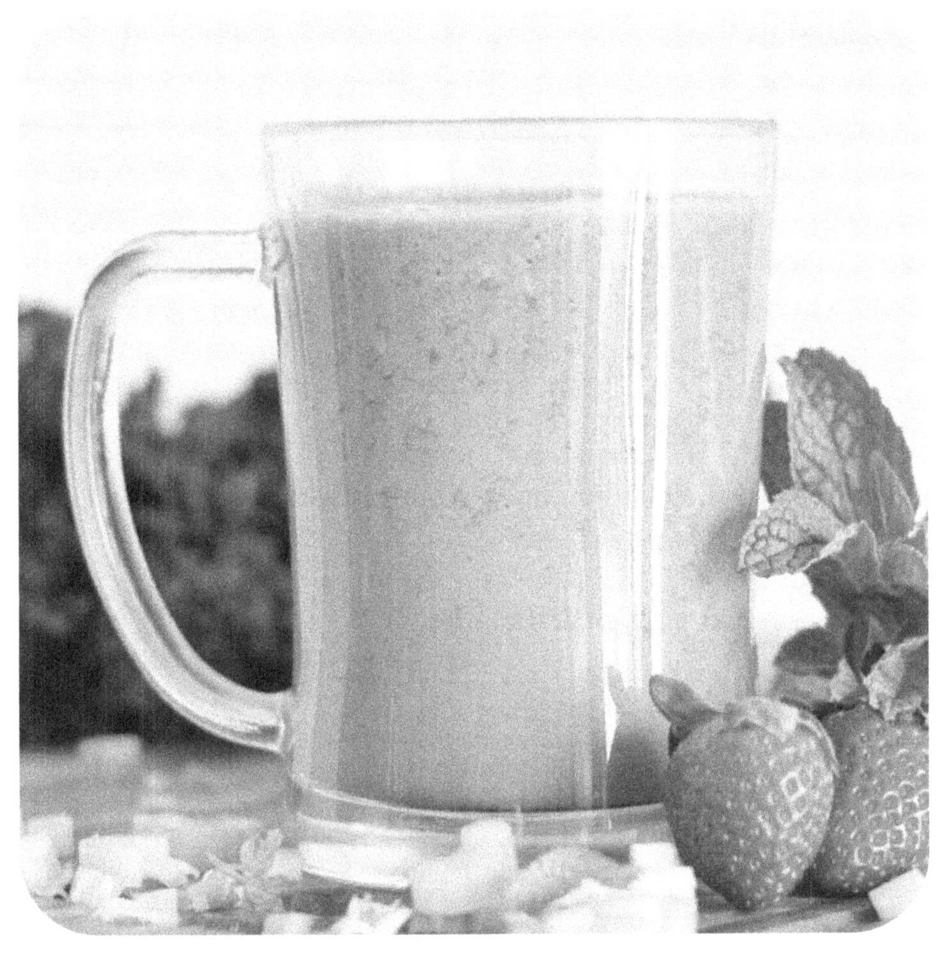

Avocado and Walnut Smoothie

Preparation Time:

10 minutes

Cooking Time:

0 minutes

Number of Servings:

2

Ingredients

- 1 ripe avocado
- 1 cup almond milk or walnut milk (choose your favorite!)
- Handful of walnuts
- Banana or berries (for extra flavor and nutrients)

Instructions

1. Add the avocado, walnuts, and your choice of fruits to a blender. Blend until smooth.
2. Pour the almond or walnut milk over the other ingredients and blend on high until everything is fully combined. You may need to pause and stir the ingredients if they get stuck.
3. Enjoy! Pour the delicious smoothie into a glass and enjoy it immediately.

Estimated Nutrition Information (per serving)

- Calories: 350 kcal

- Carbohydrates: 30g

- Protein: 7g

- Fat: 24g

- Fiber: 10g

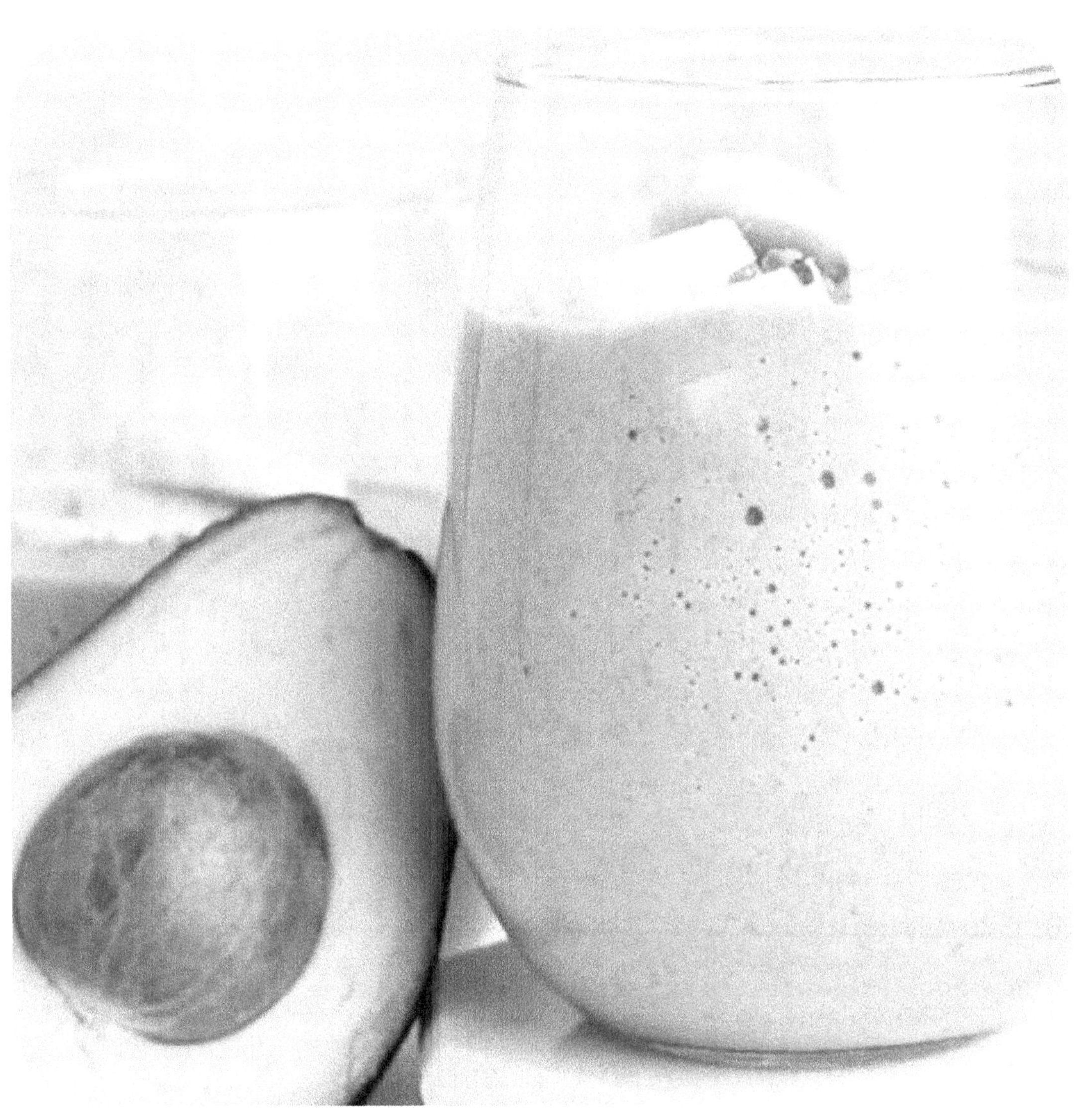

Apple Blueberry Smoothie

Preparation Time:

5 minutes

Cooking Time:

0 minutes

Number of Servings:

4

Ingredients

---

4 cups frozen blueberries

4 apples (diced)

2 cups almond milk

Instructions

1. Place the chopped apples, frozen blueberries, and almond milk in a blender. Blend until smooth. To get a completely smooth texture, you may need to pause sometimes and push the fruit down with a spoon.
2. Pour the smoothie into glasses and serve immediately.

Estimated Nutrition Information (per serving)

- Calories: 197 kcal
- Carbohydrates: 47g
- Protein: 2g

- Fiber: 8g

- Vitamin A: 178 IU

- Vitamin C: 23 mg

- Calcium: 170 mg

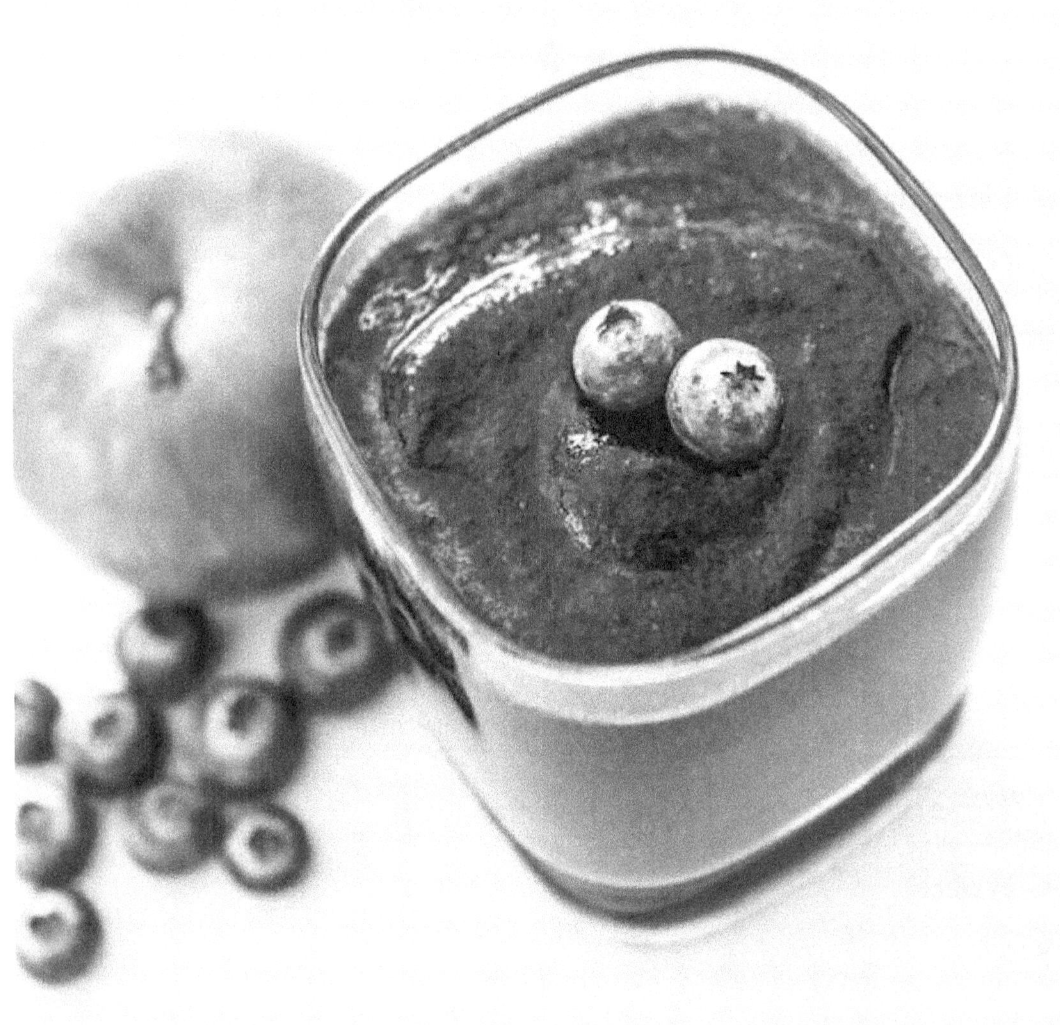

Blueberry and Coconut Smoothie

Preparation Time:

10 minutes

Cooking Time:

0 minutes

Number of Servings:

2

Ingredients

- 2 cups almond milk
- 1 cup light coconut milk
- 2 tablespoons maple syrup
- 1 cup blueberries
- 1 frozen banana

Instructions

1. Toss all your ingredients into a blender. Process everything until it is smooth and creamy.

Estimated Nutrition Information (per serving)

- Calories: 241 kcal
- Carbohydrates: 42g
- Protein: 2g
- Fat: 10g
- Fiber: 4g

- Vitamin A: 78 IU
- Vitamin C: 12 mg
- Calcium: 322 mg

Note

- Swap frozen bananas for ripe bananas and add a few ice cubes to chill your smoothie.
- Customize your smoothie by using any kind of milk you like, including plant-based options for a vegan twist.
- Want a thicker smoothie? Pour it into a bowl and add your favorite toppings for a fun and satisfying smoothie bowl experience.

Chapter 10 - Your 30-Day Meal Plan

Weekly Meal Planner

Week One

	Breakfast	Lunch	Dinner	Snacks
Day 1	Oatmeal with Peanut Butter & Banana	Grilled Chicken Salad	Grilled Shrimp and Veggie Skewers	Sliced Apples with Peanut Butter
Day 2	Scrambled Eggs with Spinach and Tomato	Grilled Salmon and Asparagus	Tomato and Lentil Soup with Spinach	No-Bake Protein Bars
Day 3	Protein Pancakes	Mixed Greens & Avocado Chicken Salad	Mini Meat Muffins with Vegetables	Sliced Apples with Almond Butter
Day 4	Greek Yogurt Berry Parfait	Chickpea Salad Sandwich	Spaghetti Squash Bolognese	Greek Yogurt with Nuts
Day 5	Easy Blueberry Biscuits	Tuna Salad Sandwich	Spaghetti Squash with Chicken, Mushrooms, Garlic, and Kale	Whipped Cottage Cheese
Day 6	Greek Yogurt Paired with Granola & Honey	Black Bean & Sweet Potato Bowl	Chicken Pesto with Spaghetti Squash	Cucumber Hummus
Day 7	Mashed Avocado and Salmon Bagel	Turkey with Avocado Salad	Oven-Baked Salmon with Sautéed Mushrooms and Steamed Broccoli	Tuna Salad with Greek Yogurt

Weekly Meal Planner

Week Two

	Breakfast	Lunch	Dinner	Snacks
Day 8	Scrambled Eggs with Mushrooms	Chicken and Veggie Tacos	Oven-Baked Salmon with Sweet Potato & Steamed Green Beans	Tuna Salad with Crackers
Day 9	Tomato & Spinach Scrambled Eggs	Grilled Zucchini and Quinoa Salad	Creamy Shrimp and Broccoli Pasta	Refreshing Liver Detox Smoothie
Day 10	Oatmeal Pancakes with Greek Yogurt	Grilled Chicken and Bean Salad	Shrimp and Veggie Cauliflower Fried Rice	5-Minute Peanut Butter and Banana Smoothie
Day 11	Whole Grain Breakfast Pancakes	Vegetables and Roasted Pork Tenderloin	Shrimp Scampi with Whole-Wheat Pasta	Carrot Cake Smoothie
Day 12	Veggie & Cheese Omelette	Mixed Greens & Avocado Chicken Salad	Grilled Shrimp and Veggie Skewers	Energizing Green Smoothie Bowl
Day 13	Greek Yogurt Berry Parfait	Chickpea Salad Sandwich	Tomato and Lentil Soup with Spinach	Protein Smoothie with Blueberries and Peanut Butter
Day 14	Oatmeal with Peanut Butter & Banana	Grilled Salmon and Asparagus	Mini Meat Muffins with Vegetables	Oatmeal and Berries Smoothie

Weekly Meal Planner

Week Three

	Breakfast	Lunch	Dinner	Snacks
Day 15	Scrambled Eggs with Spinach and Tomato	Grilled Chicken Salad	Spaghetti Squash Bolognese	Almond and Zucchini Smoothie
Day 16	Protein Pancakes	Black Bean & Sweet Potato Bowl	Spaghetti Squash with Chicken, Mushrooms, Garlic, and Kale	Avocado and Walnut Smoothie
Day 17	Greek Yogurt Berry Parfait	Tuna Salad Sandwich	Chicken Pesto with Spaghetti Squash	Apple Blueberry Smoothie
Day 18	Tomato & Spinach Scrambled Eggs	Turkey with Avocado Salad	Oven-Baked Salmon with Sautéed Mushrooms and Steamed Broccoli	Sliced Apples with Peanut Butter
Day 19	Greek Yogurt Paired with Granola & Honey	Chicken and Veggie Tacos	Oven-Baked Salmon with Sweet Potato & Steamed Green Beans	No-Bake Protein Bars
Day 20	Mashed Avocado and Salmon Bagel	Grilled Zucchini and Quinoa Salad	Creamy Shrimp and Broccoli Pasta	Sliced Apples with Almond Butter
Day 21	Scrambled Eggs with Mushrooms	Grilled Chicken and Bean Salad	Shrimp and Veggie Cauliflower Fried Rice	Greek Yogurt with Nuts

Weekly Meal Planner

Week Four

	Breakfast	Lunch	Dinner	Snacks
Day 22	Tomato & Spinach Scrambled Eggs	Vegetables and Roasted Pork Tenderloin	Shrimp Scampi with Whole-Wheat Pasta	Whipped Cottage Cheese
Day 23	Oatmeal Pancakes with Greek Yogurt	Mixed Greens & Avocado Chicken Salad	Grilled Shrimp and Veggie Skewers	Cucumber Hummus
Day 24	Whole Grain Breakfast Pancakes	Chickpea Salad Sandwich	Tomato and Lentil Soup with Spinach	Tuna Salad with Greek Yogurt
Day 25	Veggie & Cheese Omelette	Grilled Salmon and Asparagus	Mini Meat Muffins with Vegetables	Tuna Salad with Crackers
Day 26	Tomato & Spinach Scrambled Eggs	Grilled Chicken Salad	Spaghetti Squash Bolognese	Refreshing Liver Detox Smoothie
Day 27	Oatmeal with Peanut Butter & Banana	Black Bean & Sweet Potato Bowl	Spaghetti Squash with Chicken, Mushrooms, Garlic, and Kale	5-Minute Peanut Butter and Banana Smoothie
Day 28	Scrambled Eggs with Spinach and Tomato	Tuna Salad Sandwich	Chicken Pesto with Spaghetti Squash	Carrot Cake Smoothie

Weekly Meal Planner

Week Five

	Breakfast	Lunch	Dinner	Snacks
Day 29	Protein Pancakes	Turkey with Avocado Salad	Oven-Baked Salmon with Sautéed Mushrooms and Steamed Broccoli	Energizing Green Smoothie Bowl
Day 30	Mashed Avocado and Salmon Bagel	Chicken and Veggie Tacos	Oven-Baked Salmon with Sweet Potato & Steamed Green Beans	Protein Smoothie with Blueberries and Peanut Butter

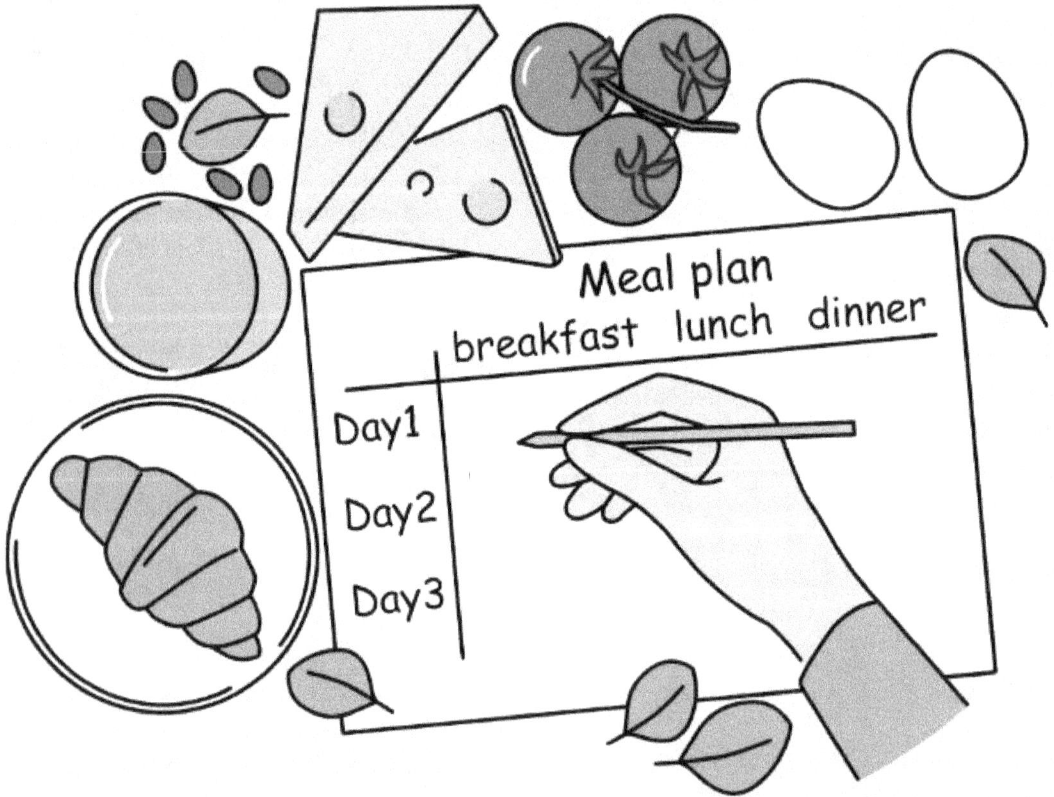

Chapter 11 - Endomorph Exercises

Endomorph body types tend to struggle with a slower metabolism and are more likely to gain weight. This doesn't mean that gaining muscle and losing weight are impossible to do; all it takes is a tailored training program. This thorough guide will help you get the most out of your workouts:

How to Exercise for Your Body Type in the Best Possible Way

To effectively manage weight and build muscle as an endomorphs, the key to success is a double play; that is cardio and strength training working together. This means focusing on workouts that help build lean muscle mass and boost metabolism. First up, cardio! We all know it burns calories and keeps your heart healthy, right? Aim for 30 to 60 minutes, 2-3 times a week. High-intensity interval training (HIIT) is a great option – short bursts of intense effort followed by recovery periods. You can also mix in some moderate-intensity cardio for variety.

Strength training, on the other hand, helps increase muscle mass, which in turn boosts metabolism and helps burn more calories even at rest. The key is to focus on compound exercises that work multiple muscle groups at once. Think squats for your legs and core, deadlifts for your entire backside, push-ups for your chest and triceps, and rows for your back and biceps. This balanced approach ensures efficient weight management and improved overall fitness.

Muscle Building

Muscle is a metabolism booster! the reason is that muscle tissue burns more calories than fat, even when you're chilling. This mean that weight training is your key to stoking that fire, helping you burn calories all day long.

Focus on complex exercises like bench presses, squats, rows, and deadlifts if you want to effectively gain muscular growth. These workouts greatly enhance powerful hormones that promote muscle growth and recruit the greatest number of muscle units. For each exercise, aim for 3–4 sets of 8–12 repetitions to maximize muscle growth and increase your rate of metabolism.

Weight Training for Endomorphs

As mentioned earlier, as an endomorph, it's time to embrace the power of weight training! Prioritize a mix of compound and isolation exercises to maximize your results. Compound exercises, such as squats, deadlifts, bench presses, and rows, engage multiple muscle groups, enhancing overall strength and muscle mass. For lower body strength, squats are your go-to, while deadlifts boost overall strength and muscle growth. Bench presses target the chest, shoulders, and triceps, and rows are perfect for strengthening the back. Don't forget leg presses to focus on the quadriceps, hamstrings, and glutes.

Incorporate these compound movements to stimulate muscle growth and increase calorie expenditure. Don't shy away from lifting heavy weights, as challenging yourself (with proper form) is key to building muscle and strength effectively. Maintain a high intensity by keeping rest periods between sets short (30-60 seconds). This approach not only boosts your metabolism but also burns more calories, helping you achieve your fitness goals.

Finding a Balance

For endomorphs, striking the right balance in your workout routine is crucial. Too much cardio can result in muscle loss, while too little can impede fat loss. Aim to incorporate 3-4 days of strength training and 2-3 days of cardio each week to effectively maintain muscle mass and promote fat burning.

Exercise Plans

The following exercise plan includes cardiovascular training, HIIT, circuit training, and flexibility exercises tailored for endomorphs.

No Equipment

Weekly Schedule

- **Day 1: Cardiovascular Training**

    o   Brisk walking for 30 minutes.

    o   Cycling for 20 minutes at a moderate pace.

- **Day 2: HIIT**

    o   Warm-up: 5 minutes of light jogging.

    o   Sprints: 30 seconds sprint, 1 minute walk (repeat 10 times).

    o   Cool-down: 5 minutes of walking and stretching.

- **Day 3: Circuit Training**

    o   Squats: 3 sets of 15 reps.

    o   Push-ups: 3 sets of 12 reps.

    o   Lunges: 3 sets of 15 reps per leg.

    o   Plank rows: 3 sets of 10 reps per side.

    o   Box step-ups: 3 sets of 12 reps per leg.

    o   Jumping jacks: 3 sets of 20 reps.

- **Day 4: Flexibility and Mobility**

    o Yoga session focusing on poses like Downward Dog, Child's Pose, and Warrior II.

    o Static stretching for all major muscle groups (hold each stretch for 30 seconds).

- **Day 5: Cardiovascular Training**

    o Running for 20 minutes at a moderate pace.

    o Swimming for 20 minutes at a steady pace.

- **Day 6: HIIT**

    o Warm-up: 5 minutes of light jogging.

    o Jump rope: 1 minute high-intensity, 1 minute rest (repeat 10 times).

    o Cool-down: 5 minutes of walking and stretching.

- **Day 7: Active Rest**

    o Light activity like a leisurely walk or a gentle yoga session.

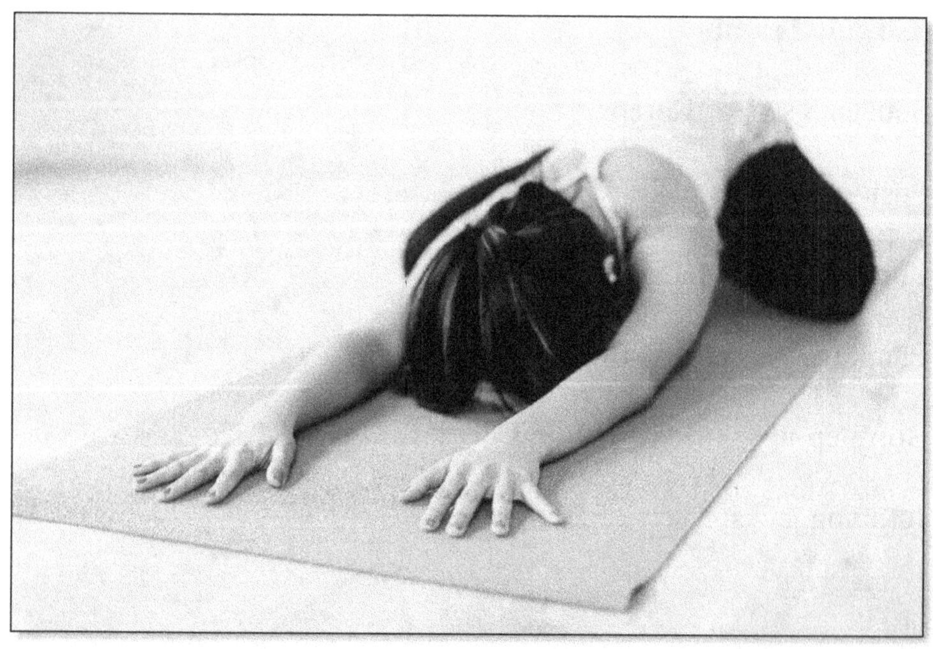

With Equipment

The exercise plan includes cardiovascular training, HIIT, weight lifting, and flexibility exercises. This comprehensive approach helps in burning calories, building muscle, and enhancing overall fitness.

Weekly Schedule

- **Day 1: Cardiovascular Training & Weight Lifting (Upper Body)**
  - **Cardio**: Brisk walking for 10 minutes as a warm-up.
  - **Weight Lifting**:
    - Bench Press: 3 sets of 12 reps
    - Bent Over Rows: 3 sets of 12 reps
    - Dumbbell Shoulder Press: 3 sets of 12 reps
    - Bicep Curls: 3 sets of 15 reps
    - Tricep Dips: 3 sets of 15 reps
  - **Cool-down**: Light stretching for upper body muscles.
- **Day 2: HIIT & Core**
  - **Warm-up**: 5 minutes of light jogging.
  - **HIIT**:
    - Sprints: 30 seconds sprint, 1-minute walk (repeat 10 times).
    - Mountain Climbers: 3 sets of 20 reps.
  - **Core**:
    - Plank: 3 sets of 1 minute.
    - Bicycle Crunches: 3 sets of 20 reps.
    - Russian Twists: 3 sets of 20 reps.

- o **Cool-down**: Light stretching focusing on core muscles.

- **Day 3: Weight Lifting (Lower Body) & Flexibility**

  - o **Warm-up**: 5 minutes of brisk walking.

  - o **Weight Lifting**:

    - Squats: 3 sets of 15 reps

    - Deadlifts: 3 sets of 12 reps

    - Leg Press: 3 sets of 12 reps

    - Calf Raises: 3 sets of 15 reps

    - Lunges: 3 sets of 15 reps per leg

  - o **Flexibility**:

    - Dynamic stretching for lower body (e.g., leg swings, hip circles).

    - Static stretching for lower body (hold each stretch for 30 seconds).

- **Day 4: Active Recovery & Light Cardio**

  - o **Light Cardio**: Cycling for 30 minutes at a moderate pace.

  - o **Flexibility**: Yoga session focusing on poses that improve flexibility and relaxation.

- **Day 5: Weight Lifting (Full Body) & HIIT**

  - o **Warm-up**: 5 minutes of light jogging.

  - o **Weight Lifting**:

    - Deadlifts: 3 sets of 10 reps

    - Overhead Press: 3 sets of 12 reps

    - Pull-ups or Lat Pulldowns: 3 sets of 10 reps

    - Dumbbell Bench Press: 3 sets of 12 reps

    - Barbell Rows: 3 sets of 12 reps

- o **HIIT**:

  - Jump Rope: 1 minute high-intensity, 1 minute rest (repeat 10 times).

- o **Cool-down**: Light stretching for full body.

- **Day 6: Cardiovascular Training & Flexibility**

  - o **Cardio**: Running for 20 minutes at a moderate pace.

  - o **Flexibility**: Pilates session focusing on core strength and flexibility.

- **Day 7: Rest or Light Activity**

  - o **Light Activity**: A leisurely walk or gentle yoga session.

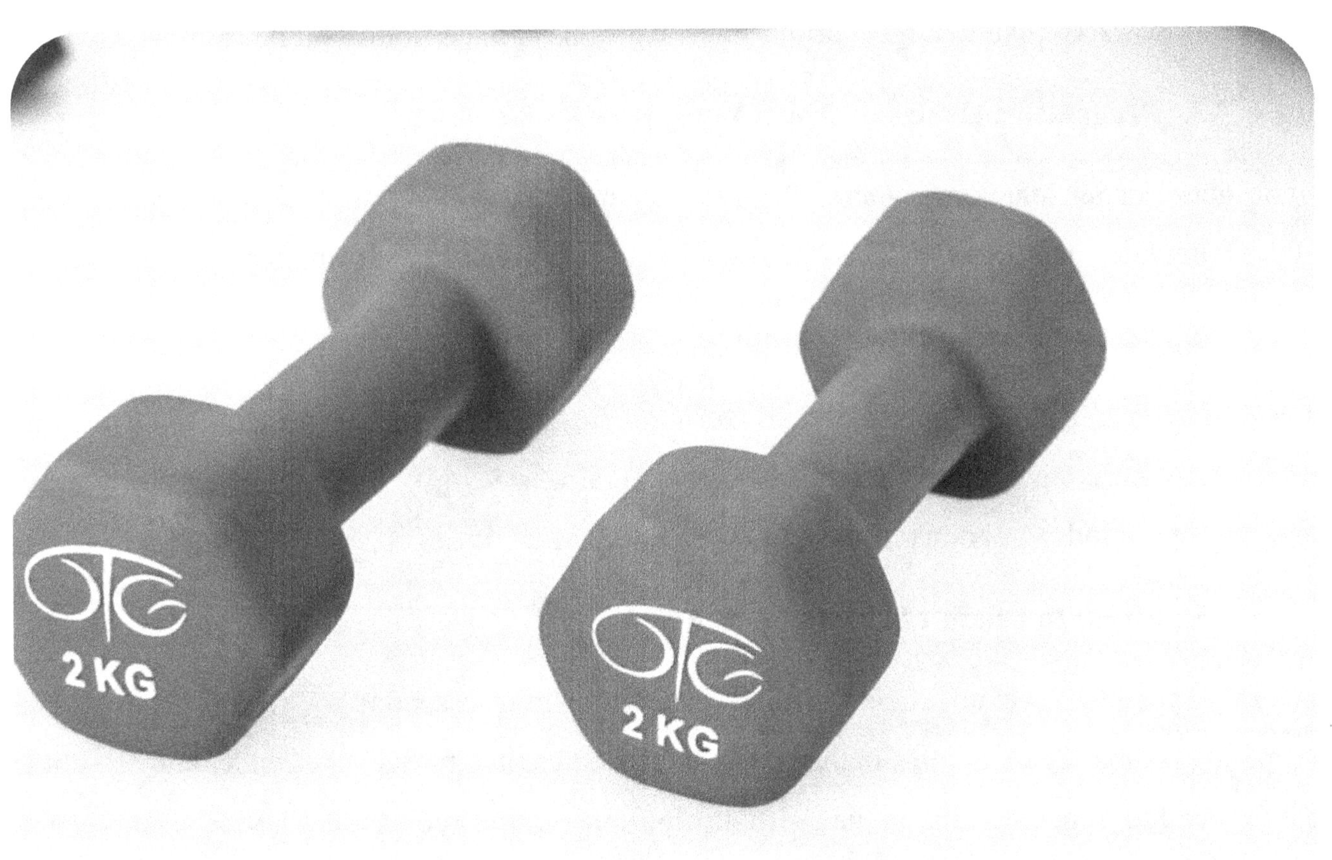

7 Workout Tips to Unleash Your Inner Fitness Machine

1. Cardio & Strength Training (The Dream Team)

Now you don't want to neglect either of these! Cardio is crucial for burning calories and heart health. Aim for 30-60 minutes 2-3 times a week, with options like the HIIT (High-Intensity Interval Training) or moderate-intensity cardio recommended in this guidebook. But don't forget the magic of strength training! Building muscle is your secret weapon. Muscle burns more calories at rest, so weight training becomes your best friend.

2. Compound Exercises: Your Muscle-Building BFFs

Focus on exercises that work for multiple muscle groups simultaneously. In our guide, we have tailored your workout plan to target various muscle groups at once from a single exercise.

3. Progressive Overload: Keep Your Muscles Guessing

As you get stronger, challenge yourself! Gradually increase weight, sets, or reps to keep your muscles stimulated and growing. This keeps your workouts fresh and your metabolism humming.

4. Rest and Heal Like a Champion

We cannot overstate the importance of rest! During recuperation, your muscles develop and mend themselves. When training the same muscle group again, try to give yourself 48 hours off. Pay attention to your body, and don't hesitate to take an additional day off if necessary.

5. Strength Doesn't Have to Be Loud

Don't be scared to give up on ego-lifting! Proper form is essential to avoiding injury and maximizing results. The workouts in this guide have been created to fit every gender and age alike. but it's crucial to remember that in the (**with equipment section**) you should not be afraid to start with lighter weights and focus on controlled movements.

6. Fuel Your Body with the Right Food

What you eat matters! Focus on a balanced diet that includes lean protein for muscle building, complex carbs for energy, and healthy fats to keep you satisfied. Our recipes in this diet book have been portioned to get you the best macronutrient levels for your body type. Remember, nutrition is half the battle!

7. **Find Your Fitness Groove (Never Lose Motivation)**

Consistency is key! Find activities you enjoy, whether it's hitting the gym, joining a fitness class, or training outdoors. You're more likely to stick with it long-term when you have fun.

Chapter 12 - Top FAQs about Endomorph Diet and Exercise Plan

How does metabolism influence weight loss for endomorphs?

Endomorphs typically have a slower metabolism, making their bodies more efficient at storing energy as fat. This metabolic trait makes it easier for endomorphs to gain weight and more challenging to lose it. Even when consuming the same diet as individuals with different body types, endomorphs are more likely to retain excess fat.

What is the endomorph diet, and how does it suit this body type?

The endomorph diet is specifically designed to enhance metabolism and effectively manage body weight by emphasizing high protein and lower carbohydrate intake. It involves a balanced distribution of macronutrients and prioritizes foods that promote satiety and energy without causing blood sugar spikes.

As an endomorph how do calories affect my weight gain and loss?

Endomorphs are particularly sensitive to calorie consumption, often needing to carefully monitor their food intake to avoid consuming more calories than they burn. Excess calorie intake can lead to increased fat storage, necessitating meticulous dietary management for weight control.

How can endomorphs monitor their calorie intake to lose weight effectively?

Endomorphs can effectively monitor their calorie intake by measuring food portions and tracking daily caloric consumption. This practice helps ensure they do not exceed their caloric needs, facilitating better weight management.

What advantages does exercise offer for endomorphs?

Exercise is essential for endomorphs as it helps build muscle and boost metabolism. A well-rounded workout plan for endomorphs should include both cardio exercises to increase daily calorie expenditure and weight training to promote muscle growth.

What is the best endomorph diet plan?

The optimal diet for endomorphs involves reducing calorie intake while increasing the consumption of lean proteins, healthy fats (such as omega fatty acids), and low carbohydrates. This balanced approach helps manage weight and support overall health.

What foods should endomorphs avoid?

While endomorphs should focus on consuming lean proteins, complex carbohydrates, and healthy fats they should limit their intake of refined carbohydrates, processed foods, and foods high in added sugars and trans fats to avoid unnecessary weight gain.

What is the nutrient distribution for an endomorph diet?

A typical endomorph diet should aim for a macronutrient distribution of approximately 30% carbohydrates, 35% protein, and 35% fat. This balance supports metabolic health and weight management.

What should my daily liquid (water) intake be like?

The U.S. National Academies of Sciences, Engineering, and Medicine recommend that men consume about 15.5 cups (3.7 liters) of fluids daily, while women should aim for about 11.5 cups (2.7 liters) of fluids each day.

What is an endomorph body type?

Endomorphs generally have softer, curvier bodies with wide waists and hips, and larger bones. They may carry more weight in their hips, thighs, and lower abdomen, often possessing higher amounts of both body fat and muscle.

Is it possible to change your body type?

While genetics largely determine your body type, you can improve and enhance your body shape through proper nutrition and targeted exercise. Each body type requires a tailored approach to fitness and diet to achieve the best results.

What are the characteristics of an endomorph body type?

Endomorphs often have slower metabolisms, making fat storage easier and weight loss more challenging. They might also have a tendency towards food cravings, comfort eating, and a more sedentary lifestyle.

As an endomorph, what is the best workout for me?

The most effective workout for endomorphs combines resistance or strength training with cardio exercises. Cardio helps increase daily calorie burn, while resistance training supports muscle development.

What are some of the best strength training exercises for endomorphs?

Effective strength training exercises for endomorphs include kettlebell swings, step-ups, burpees, power cleans, and deadlifts. These exercises help build muscle and improve overall fitness.

How often should endomorphs exercise?

Endomorphs should aim to exercise 2-3 times per week, incorporating two full-body resistance training sessions and three cardio-focused workouts for optimal results.

What additional advice is there for endomorphs trying to lose weight?

Endomorphs can achieve successful weight loss by practicing balanced nutrition, portion control, regular strength training, and maintaining a positive attitude. Consulting a dietitian for personalized dietary advice can also be beneficial.

I think I have reached a weight-loss plateau and I'm no longer losing weight. What should I do?

Hitting a weight-loss plateau may indicate that you've exhausted the weight-loss potential of your current diet and exercise plan. To continue losing weight, you'll need to adjust your weight-loss strategy, possibly by modifying your diet or increasing exercise intensity.

Recipe Index List

Breakfast

Lunch

7. Grilled Zucchini and Quinoa Salad - 61

8. Mixed Greens & Avocado Chicken Salad - 48

9. Tuna Salad Sandwich - 52

10. Turkey with Avocado Salad - 56

11. Vegetables and Roasted Pork Tenderloin - 67

Dinner

1. Chicken Pesto with Spaghetti Squash - 82

2. Creamy Shrimp and Broccoli Pasta - 90

3. Grilled Shrimp and Veggie Skewers - 69

4. Mini Meat Muffins with Vegetables - 74

5. Oven-Baked Salmon with Sautéed Mushrooms and Steamed Broccoli - 84

6. Oven-Baked Salmon with Sweet Potato & Steamed Green Beans - 87

7. Shrimp and Veggie Cauliflower Fried Rice - 92

8. Shrimp Scampi with Whole-Wheat Pasta - 94

9. Spaghetti Squash Bolognese - 76

10. Spaghetti Squash with Chicken, Mushrooms, Garlic, And Kale - 79

11. Tomato and Lentil Soup with Spinach - 72

Snacks

1. 5-Minute Peanut Butter and Banana Smoothie - 114

2. Almond and Zucchini Smoothie - 124

3. Apple Blueberry Smoothie - 128

4. Avocado and Walnut Smoothie - 126

5. Blueberry and Coconut Smoothie - 130

6. Carrot Cake Smoothie - 116

7. Cucumber Hummus - 106

8. Energizing Green Smoothie Bowl - 118

9. Greek Yogurt with Nuts - 102

10. No-Bake Protein Bars - 98

11. Oatmeal and Berries Smoothie - 122

12. Protein Smoothie with Blueberries and Peanut Butter - 120

13. Refreshing Liver Detox Smoothie - 112

14. Sliced Apples with Almond Butter - 100

15. Sliced Apples with Peanut Butter - 96

16. Tuna Salad with Crackers - 110

17. Tuna Salad with Greek Yogurt - 108

18. Whipped Cottage Cheese - 104